Essentials of Atrial Fibrillation

Essentials of Atrial Fibrillation

Yee Guan Yap
Head and Associate Professor of Cardiology
Putra University, Selangor, Malaysia
and
Consultant Interventional Cardiologist
Prince Court Medical Centre, Kuala Lumpur, Malaysia

A John Camm
Professor of Clinical Cardiology
Division of Clinical Sciences
St George's University of London, London, UK
and
Honorary Consultant Cardiologist
St George's Hospital, London, UK

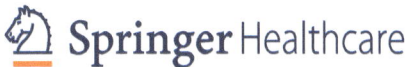

Published by Springer Healthcare,236 Gray's Inn Road, London, WC1X 8HB, UK

www.springerhealthcare.com

First published 2010
Revised edition 2014

British Library Cataloguing-in-Publication Data.

A catalogue record for this book is available from the British Library.

ISBN 978 1 85873 438 5

Although every effort has been made to ensure that drug doses and other information are presented accurately in this publication, the ultimate responsibility rests with the prescribing physician. Neither the publisher nor the authors can be held responsible for errors or for any consequences arising from the use of the information contained herein. Any product mentioned in this publication should be used in accordance with the prescribing information prepared by the manufacturers. No claims or endorsements are made for any drug or compound at present under clinical investigation.

Project editor: Anne Carty and Katrina Dorn
Designer: Joe Harvey
Artworker: Sissan Mollerfors
Production: Marina Maher
Printed inGreat Britainby Latimer Trend

Contents

Author biographies

Yee Guan Yap, BMedSci(Nottm), MBBS(Nottm), MD(Lond), FRCP(Glasg), FRCP(Edin), FRCP(Lond), FESC, FSCAI, FAHA, FACC, is the Head of the Department of Medicine and Unit of Cardiology and an Associate Professor of Cardiology and Medicine at Putra University, Malaysia. He is also a Consultant Interventional Cardiologist at the Prince Court Medical Centre, Kuala Lumpur, Malaysia. He graduated with BMedSci(Hons) and MBBS from the University of Nottingham, UK, and subsequently obtained his postgraduate Doctorate of Medicine (MD) degree from the University of London for his research thesis on risk stratification for sudden cardiac death after myocardial infarction. He received his postgraduate subspeciality training in Cardiology and Internal Medicine at a large busy tertiary cardiac centre in St. George's Hospital, London, UK. Upon completion of his postgraduate training, he was awarded the United Kingdom Postgraduate Medical Education and Training Board Certification in Cardiology and the European Board for the Specialty of Cardiology Diploma of European Cardiologist. He became an accredited and registered consultant specialist in cardiology with the UK General Medical Council before returning to Malaysia in 2005 to take up his current position.

Dr Yap's main clinical interests are interventional cardiology, device therapies, including biventricular pacemaker and implantable cardiac defibrillator therapies (ICD), and structural heart disease. His main research interest is risk stratification of post-myocardial infarction patients who are at risk of sudden cardiac death for ICD implantation and acquired long QT syndrome. He was a recipient of the British Heart Foundation Research Fellowship in 1997. He has published extensively in cardiology in international medical journals, as well as contributing book chapters and authoring books. He lectures widely at national and international meetings and conferences and is a regular referee for a number of international medical journals.

A John Camm, BSc(Lond), MBBS(Lond), MD(Lond), FMed Sci, FRCP(Edin), FRCP(Lond), FESC, FAHA, FACC, FHRS, graduated from Guy's Hospital, London and pursued a career in cardiology at St. Bartholomew's Hospital. In 1986, he moved to the British Heart Foundation Chair of Clinical Cardiology at St George's University of London. Currently, John Camm is professor of clinical cardiology at St George's University of London and honorary consultant cardiologist at St George's Hospital in London, United Kingdom.

Professor Camm's research interests include clinical electrocardiology, clinical cardiac electrophysiology, cardiac arrhythmias, implantable devices for rhythm control, risk stratification for sudden death in patients with ischemic heart disease, for thromboembolism in patients with atrial fibrillation, and for ventricular arrhythmia in patients with cardiomyopathy and channelopathy, adverse cardiovascular events in new and old drugs, and anticoagulation.

Professor Camm is past chairman of the European Society of Cardiology Working Group on Cardiac Arrhythmias (now European Heart Rhythm Association), past president of the British Pacing and Electrophysiology Group (now Heart Rhythm UK), past council member of the Royal College of Physicians, and past trustee of the North American Society of Pacing and Electrophysiology (now Heart Rhythm Society) and the American College of Cardiology. Professor Camm is also a former chairman of the Joint Cardiology Committee (Royal College of Physicians of London) and past president of the British Cardiovascular Society. Professor Camm holds the European Society of Cardiology Gold Medal.

Professor Camm is currently a board member of the European Heart Rhythm Association, the World Society of Arrhythmias, and the Drug Safety Research Unit. He is president of the Arrhythmia Alliance, and founder and trustee of the Atrial Fibrillation Association. He is editor-in-chief of *Clinical Cardiology* and *Europace* and an editor of the *European Heart Journal* and the *European Society of Cardiology Textbook of Cardiovascular Medicine*.

Chapter 1

Epidemiology of atrial fibrillation

Prevalence and incidence of atrial fibrillation

Atrial fibrillation (AF; Figure 1.1) is the most common cardiac arrhythmia that clinicians encounter in their daily clinical practice. AF affects 1.0–1.5% of the population in the developed world [1,2]. Currently, in the USA, approximately 3 million people have a diagnosis of AF and, based on the census, this number may rise to 12 million by 2050 [3].

The prevalence and incidence of AF increases sharply with advancing age. The prevalence of AF rises from 0.7% in the age group 55–59 years to 17.8% in those aged 85 years and over [4]. The overall incidence for AF is 9.9/1000 person-years [4], and the incidence in the group aged 55–59 years is 1.1/1000 person-years, which rises to 20.7/1000 person-years in the group aged 80–84 years and stabilizes in those aged 85 years and above. Of note, 70% of AF patients are aged between 65 and 85 years and, overall, 84% are older than 65 years [5].

In the Framingham study, the lifetime risk for the development of AF was one in four for men and women aged 40 years and older [6]. The data from Europe showed a similar lifetime risk of developing AF after the age of 55 years: 23.8% in men and 22.2% in women [4]. AF is 12–20 times more common in people aged 80–85 years compared with individuals aged 50–60 years [4,6].

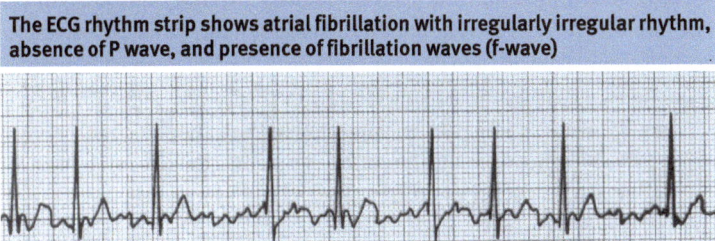

The ECG rhythm strip shows atrial fibrillation with irregularly irregular rhythm, absence of P wave, and presence of fibrillation waves (f-wave)

Figure 1.1 **The ECG rhythm strip shows atrial fibrillation with irregularly irregular rhythm, absence of discrete P waves, and presence of fibrillation waves (f-waves).**

© Springer Healthcare 2014
Y.G. Yap and A.J. Camm, *Essentials of Atrial Fibrillation*,
DOI 10.1007/978-1-907673-98-6_1

Mortality, morbidity, and quality of life in atrial fibrillation

AF can cause distressing palpitations and shortness of breath. It can also precipitate ischemic syndromes and heart failure. Patients with AF have a threefold increased risk of congestive cardiac failure [7]. Heart failure promotes AF, which in turn aggravates heart failure. Individuals with either condition who develop the other condition share a poor prognosis.

AF is also associated with up to twice the rate of total mortality and cardiovascular death compared with patients in normal sinus rhythm, and is linked to the severity of underlying heart disease [8,9]. The risk of stroke is increased fivefold with AF [10]. The annual incidence of ischemic stroke is 5% among people with non-valvular AF, two to seven times that of people without AF [1]. Approximately one in six ischemic strokes is associated with AF, and most result from embolization of left atrial appendage thrombi [11]. The clinical significance of AF-related strokes is due to the higher mortality, greater disability, increased costs, and increasing incidence of recurrent stroke within 1 year [11]. Non-valvular AF-related stroke causes a substantial loss of life years. A nationwide, population-based, follow-up study of patients aged 40–80 years with incidental hospital diagnosis of AF or atrial flutter, has examined the mean loss of life years attributable to incident stroke within 20 years of a first diagnosis of AF. The mean loss was up to 10 years, though the loss was frequently less than 5 years [12]. Women, younger patients, and those who had a stroke early after the diagnosis of AF had the largest number of lost life years. The relative loss of life years was up to 90% of the estimated expected remaining lifetime without stroke within 20 years of the diagnosis of AF. Elderly people had the highest relative loss.

AF also results in more hospital admissions than any other arrhythmia. The number of AF-related hospitalizations across the world almost tripled in 2000 compared with two decades previously [13,14]. Among UK hospital admissions, AF is present in 3–6% of acute medical admissions [15,16].

Quality of life is impaired in patients with AF compared with healthy people. The presence of complaints of AF at baseline, a short duration of AF, and the presence of sinus rhythm (SR) at the end of follow-up were associated with improvement in quality of life in one study of the influence of rate control and rhythm control [17]. Treatment strategy (rhythm control vs rate control) does not affect quality of life [17,18]. However, patients with symptoms related to AF may benefit from rhythm control if SR can be maintained [17,19]. The improvement in quality of life also correlates with an improvement in exercise performance [20].

Social economics of atrial fibrillation

Treatment of AF represents a significant healthcare burden, especially when treating inpatients. In 2001, in three federally funded databases in the USA [21], the total annual costs for treatment of AF were estimated at US$6.65 billion, including:

- US$2.93 billion (44%) for hospitalizations with a principal discharge diagnosis of AF
- US$1.95 billion (29%) for the incremental inpatient cost of AF as a comorbid diagnosis
- US$1.53 billion (23%) for outpatient treatment of AF
- US$235 million (4%) for prescription drugs.

In all circumstances, AF was a significant contributor to hospital cost.

Within the US healthcare system, after initial diagnosis, patients with AF treated with traditional therapies incur US$4000–5000 in annual direct healthcare costs, with about half of these costs attributable to inpatient care. There is a substantial variation in annual costs according to the clinical course of the AF. Patients with permanent AF from the outset have the lowest resource utilization and costs. Costs are markedly higher in patients with multiple AF recurrences, with each recurrence increasing annual costs by a mean of US$1600 [22]. The AFFIRM analysis demonstrated that patients randomized to pharmacologic rhythm control had greater resource utilization and higher costs than patients randomized to rate control (US$25,600 vs US$20,500 over 4.6 years) [23]. Paradoxically, in France, patients with persistent/permanent AF had significantly higher hospitalization rates and costs than patients with paroxysmal AF (€3579 vs €2586 euros), with the cost of hospital care accounting for roughly half the total costs [24].

The area of greatest variation in costs for patients with AF is hospital care, with some of this cost being wasteful. Some of the treatments traditionally provided in hospitals can be safely delivered on an outpatient basis at much less expense. Institution of a practice guideline has been shown to be safe, effective, and cost-saving, with an average decrease in 30-day total direct healthcare costs of approximately US$1400 per patient [25], mainly due to a decrease in the rate of hospital admission (from 74% to 38%), with no differences in return visits to emergency departments or hospital readmission within 30 days, stroke, or death. Thus, there should be widespread adoption of AF practice guidelines.

The evidence to date has suggested that the traditional way of managing AF (with drug therapy and cardioversion) is expensive. For patients with minimal or no symptoms from their AF, rate control and anticoagulation are probably an acceptable clinical strategy [23,26]. They are also very likely to be the least expensive, unless a highly successful rhythm control strategy can be shown to prevent strokes and/or reduce the need for chronic anticoagulation [22,27].

References

1. Fuster V, Rydén LE, Cannom DS, American College of Cardiology Foundation/American Heart Association Task Force, et al. 2011 ACCF/AHA/HRS focused updates incorporated into the ACC/AHA/ESC 2006 guidelines for the management of patients with atrial fibrillation: a report of the American College of Cardiology Foundation/American Heart Association Task Force on practice guidelines. *Circulation*. 2011;123:e269-e367.

2. Centers for Disease Control and Prevention (CDC). Atrial Fibrillation Fact Sheet. CDC website. www.cdc.gov/dhdsp/data_statistics/fact_sheets/docs/fs_atrial_fibrillation.pdf. Accessed March 11, 2013.

3. Kannel WB, Benjamin EJ. Status of the epidemiology of atrial fibrillation. *Med Clin North Am*. 2008;92:17-40.

4. Heeringa J, van der Kuip DA, Hofman A, et al. Prevalence, incidence and lifetime risk of atrial fibrillation: the Rotterdam study. *Eur Heart J*. 2006;27:949-953.

5. Lip GYH, Lalukota K. Atrial fibrillation. *J R Coll Physicians Edin*. 2007;37:238-343.

6. Lloyd-Jones DM, Wang TJ, Leip EP, et al. Lifetime risk for development of atrial fibrillation: the Framingham Heart Study. *Circulation*. 2004;110:1042-1046.

7. Gottdiener JS, Arnold AM, Aurigemma GP, et al. Predictors of congestive heart failure in the elderly: the cardiovascular Health Study. *J Am Coll Cardiol*. 2000;35:1628-1637.

8. Kannel WB, Abbott RD, Savage DD, McNamara PM. Epidemiologic features of atrial fibrillation: the Framingham study. *N Engl J Med*. 1982;306:1018-1022.

9. Krahn DA, Manfreda J, Tate BR, Mathewson FAL, Cuddy TE. Prognosis of atrial fibrillation in men. Manitoba Follow-up Study (MFUS) (abstr). *J Am Coll Cardiol*. 1993;21:478A.

10. Wolf PA, Abbot R, Kennel W. Atrial fibrillation as an independent risk factor for stroke: the Framingham study. *Stroke*. 1991;22:983-988.

11. Saveliena I, Camm AJ. Atrial fibrillation – all change! *Clin Med*. 2007;7:374-379.

12. Frost L, Andersen LV, Johnson SP, Mortensen LS. Lost life years attributable to stroke among patients with non-valvular atrial fibrillation: a nationwide population-based follow-up study. *Neuroepidemiology*. 2007;29:59-65.

13. Stewart S, MacIntyre K, MacLeod MM, et al. Trends in hospital activity, morbidity, and case fatality related to atrial fibrillation in Scotland, 1986–1996. *Eur Heart J*. 2001;22:693-701.

14. Wattigney WA, Mensah GA, Croft JB. Increasing trends in hospitalisation for atrial fibrillation in the United States, 1985 through 1999: implications for primary prevention. *Circulation*. 2003;108:711-716.

15. Lip GY, Tean KN, Dunn FG. Treatment of atrial fibrillation in a district general hospital. *Br Heart J*. 1994;71:92-95.

16. Zarifis J, Beevers G, Lip GY. Acute admissions with atrial fibrillation in a British multiracial hospital population. *Br J Clin Pract*. 1997;51:91-96.

17. Hagens VE, Ranchor AV, Van Sonderen E, et al. RACE Study Group. Effect of rate or rhythm control on quality of life in persistent atrial fibrillation. Results from the Rate Control Versus Electrical Cardioversion (RACE) Study. *J Am Coll Cardiol*. 2004;43:241-247.

18. Jenkins LS, Brodsky M, Schron E, et al. Quality of life in atrial fibrillation: the Atrial Fibrillation Follow-up Investigation of Rhythm Management (AFFIRM) study. *Am Heart J*. 2005;149:112-120.

19. Dorian P, Paquette M, Newman D, et al. Quality of life improves with treatment in the Canadian Trial of Atrial Fibrillation. *Am Heart J*. 2002;143:984-990.

20. Singh SN, Tang XC, Singh BN, et al. SAFE-T Investigators. Quality of life and exercise performance in patients in sinus rhythm versus persistent atrial fibrillation. Veterans Affairs Cooperative Studies Program Substudy. *J Am Coll Cardiol*. 2006;48:721-730.

21. Coyne KS, Paramore C, Grandy S, Mercader M, Reynolds M, Zimetbaum P. Assessing the direct costs of treating nonvalvular atrial fibrillation in the United States. *Value Health*. 2006;9:348-356.

22. Reynolds MR, Essebag V, Zimetbaum P, Cohen DJ. Healthcare resource utilization and costs associated with recurrent episodes of atrial fibrillation: The FRACTAL registry. *J Cardiovasc Electrophysiol.* 2007;18:628-633.
23. Marshall DA, Levy AR, Vidaillet H, et al. Cost-effectiveness of rhythm versus rate control in atrial fibrillation. *Ann Intern Med.* 2004;141:653-661.
24. Le Heuzey JY, Paziaud O, Piot O, et al. Cost of care distribution in atrial fibrillation patients: The COCAF study. *Am Heart J.* 2004;147:121-126.
25. Zimetbaum P, Reynolds MR, Ho KK, et al. Impact of a practice guideline for patients with atrial fibrillation on medical resource utilization and costs. *Am J Cardiol.* 2003;92:677-681.
26. Van Gelder IC, Hagens VE, Bosker HA, et al. for the Rate Control versus Electrical Cardioversion for Persistent Atrial Fibrillation Study Group. A comparison of rate control and rhythm control in patients with recurrent persistent atrial fibrillation. *N Engl J Med.* 2002;347:1834-1840.
27. Wyse DG, Waldo AL, DiMarco JP, et al. A comparison of rate control and rhythm control in patients with atrial fibrillation. *N Engl J Med.* 2002;347:1825-1833.

Chapter 2

Pathogenesis of atrial fibrillation

Mechanism of atrial fibrillation

The mechanism of atrial fibrillation (AF) is still debatable. Several mechanisms have been proposed and seen in a variety of animal models. A traditional mechanism theory has suggested that AF is maintained by multiple migrating wavelets of re-entrant atrial activation. During AF, the atria contract at a rate of 350–900 beats/min, conducting to the ventricles at a rate of 90–170 beats/min. The wavelet collisions cause chaotic re-excitation and re-excite the multiple propagating wavelets [1,2].

It has been shown that AF is probably triggered by a rapidly firing focal source (usually in the superior pulmonary veins, but it can be in other pulmonary veins, the ligament of Marshall, the atrial septum, the superior vena cava, or right atrium) . The rapidly firing foci may stimulate multiple wavelet re-entry within the atrial substrate or engage a spiral or rotor for of re-entry [3-5]. Moreover, atrial interstitial fibrosis has also been shown to increase AF vulnerability by creating a substrate for intra-atrial re-entry circuit (intracellular scar) that promotes AF [6]. Atrial interstitial fibrosis is increased with age in humans and in congestive heart failure (CHF).

Autonomic influences in atrial fibrillation

The balance between sympathetic and vagal influences plays an important role in the initiation and prediction of AF. Vagal predominance has been observed in the minutes preceding the onset of AF in some patients with structurally normal hearts, while in others there is a shift toward sympathetic predominance [7,8]. Although certain patients can be characterized in terms of a vagal or an adrenergic form of AF, these cases likely represent the extremes of either influence [9]. In general, vagally mediated AF occurs at night or after meals, while adrenergically induced AF typically occurs during the daytime [10]. In patients with vagally mediated AF (the more common

© Springer Healthcare 2014
Y.G. Yap and A.J. Camm, *Essentials of Atrial Fibrillation*,
DOI 10.1007/978-1-907673-98-6_2

form), adrenergic-blocking drugs, or digitalis, sometimes worsen symptoms. For AF of the adrenergic type, β-blockers are the initial treatment of choice.

Risk factors and causes of atrial fibrillation

The risk factors and causes of AF can be broadly divided into several categories: reversible causes, cardiac, non-cardiac, autonomic, and familial [11].

Reversible causes of atrial fibrillation

AF may be related to acute temporary causes, such as an alcohol binge (holiday heart syndrome), thyrotoxicosis, surgery (cardiac or non-cardiac), electrocution, acute myocardial infarction, pericarditis, myocarditis, pulmonary embolism or other pulmonary diseases (eg, pneumonia), hyperthyroidism, and pheochromocytoma. In such cases, successful treatment of the underlying condition often eliminates AF. AF is also very common after surgery, including cardiac, pulmonary, or esophageal surgery.

Obesity, sleep apnea, and metabolic syndrome has also been linked to the development of AF, probably as a result of left atrial dilation associated with increased body mass index. Weight loss has been linked to regression of left atrial enlargement [12,13].

If atrial fibrillation is provoked by a so-called transient cause, it is more likely that these patients will have subsequent recurrences of the arrhythmias, provoked by similar or other factors.

Atrial fibrillation associated with heart disease

Mitral valve disease (including mitral stenosis and regurgitation and mitral valve prolapse), tricuspid valve disease, coronary artery disease, heart failure, and hypertension, particularly when left ventricular hypertrophy (LVH) is present, are associated with AF. In addition, AF may be associated with hypertrophic cardiomyopathy, dilated cardiomyopathy, or atrial septal defect in adults. Other cardiac causes include:
- infiltrative restrictive cardiomyopathies (eg, amyloidosis, hemochromatosis, and endomyocardial fibrosis);
- cardiac tumors; and
- constrictive pericarditis (from tuberculosis).

Other conditions that have been associated with a high incidence of AF include cor pulmonale.

In the setting of acute myocardial infarction, the development of AF carries a worse prognosis compared with pre-infarct AF or sinus rhythm [14,15]. When AF is associated with atrial flutter, Wolff–Parkinson–White syndrome, or atrioventricular nodal re-entrant tachycardia, treatment of the underlying primary arrhythmia reduces or eliminates the incidence of recurrent AF [16].

Atrial fibrillation without associated heart disease
Approximately 30–45% of cases of paroxysmal AF and 20–25% of cases of persistent AF occur in young patients without identifiable underlying disease (lone AF) [17,18]. AF can present as an isolated or familial arrhythmia, although a causal underlying disease may appear over time [19]. AF may also occur in the elderly without underlying heart disease as a result of the changes in cardiac structure and function that accompany aging, such as increased myocardial stiffness.

Familial atrial fibrillation
Familial AF, defined as lone AF running in a family, is more common than previously recognized. The likelihood of developing AF is increased among the children of patients with AF, suggesting a familial susceptibility to the arrhythmia. However, the mechanisms associated with genetic transmission are not necessarily electrical, because the relationship has also been seen in patients with a family history of hypertension, diabetes, or heart failure [20]. The molecular defects responsible for familial AF are largely unknown. Specific chromosomal loci associated with AF in some families suggest distinct genetic mutations [21,22]. AF is more common is some channelopathies such as Brugada syndrome, short and long QT syndromes.

References
1. Allessie M, Lammers WJEP, Bonke, FIM, Hollen, J. Experimental evaluation of Moe's multiple wavelet hypothesis of atrial fibrillation. In: Zipes DP, Jalife J (eds), *Cardiac Electrophysiology and Arrhythmias*. Orlando, FL: Grune & Stratton Inc.; 1985:265-275.
2. Moe GKRW, Abildskov JA. A computer model of atrial fibrillation. *Am Heart J*. 1964;67:200-220.
3. Haissaguerre M, Jais P, Shah DC, et al. Spontaneous initiation of atrial fibrillation by ectopic beats originating in the pulmonary veins. *N Engl J Med*. 1998;339:659-666.
4. Mandapati R, Skanes A, Chen J, et al. Stable microreentrant sources as a mechanism of atrial fibrillation in the isolated sheep heart. *Circulation*. 2000;101:194-199.
5. Skanes AC, Mandapati R, Berenfeld O, et al. Spatiotemporal periodicity during atrial fibrillation in the isolated sheep heart. *Circulation*. 1998;98:1236-1248.
6. Everett IV TH, Olgin JE. Atrial fibrosis and the mechanisms of atrial fibrillation. *Heart Rhythm*. 2007;4(3 suppl):S24-S27.
7. Fioranelli M, Piccoli M, Mileto GM, et al. Analysis of heart rate variability five minutes before the onset of paroxysmal atrial fibrillation. *Pacing Clin Electrophysiol*. 1999;22:743-749.
8. Herweg B, Dalal P, Nagy B, et al. Power spectral analysis of heart period variability of preceding sinus rhythm before initiation of paroxysmal atrial fibrillation. *Am J Cardiol*. 1998;82:869-874.
9. Coumel P. Neural aspects of paroxysmal atrial fibrillation. In: Falk RH, Podrid PJ (eds), *Atrial Fibrillation: Mechanisms and Management*. New York: Raven Press, 1992:109-125.

10. Maisel WH. Autonomic modulation preceding the onset of atrial fibrillation. *J Am Coll Cardiol*. 2003;42:1269-1270.
11. Fuster V, Rydén LE, Cannom DS, American College of Cardiology Foundation/American Heart Association Task Force, et al. 2011 ACCF/AHA/HRS focused updates incorporated into the ACC/AHA/ESC 2006 guidelines for the management of patients with atrial fibrillation: a report of the American College of Cardiology Foundation/American Heart Association Task Force on practice guidelines. *Circulation*. 2011;123:e269-e367.
12. Frost L, Hune LJ, Vestergaard P. Overweight and obesity as risk factors for atrial fibrillation or flutter: the Danish Diet, Cancer, and Health Study. *Am J Med* 2005;118:489-495.
13. Wang TJ, Parise H, Levy D, et al. Obesity and the risk of new-onset atrial fibrillation. *JAMA*. 2004;292:2471-2477.
14. Rathore SS, Berger AK, Weinfurt KP, et al. Acute myocardial infarction complicated by atrial fibrillation in the elderly: prevalence and outcomes. *Circulation*. 2000;101:969-974.
15. Goldberg RJ, Yarzebski J, Lessard D, et al. Recent trends in the incidence rates of and death rates from atrial fibrillation complicating initial acute myocardial infarction: a community-wide perspective. *Am Heart J*. 2002;143:519-527.
16. Prystowsky EN. Tachycardia-induced-tachycardia: a mechanism of initiation of atrial fibrillation. In: DiMarco JP, Prystowsky EN (eds), *Atrial Arrhythmias: State of the Art*. Armonk, NY: Futura; 1995.
17. Evans W, Swann P. Lone auricular fibrillation. *Br Heart J*. 1954;16:194.
18. Brand FN, Abbott RD, Kannel WB, et al. Characteristics and prognosis of lone atrial fibrillation. 30-year follow-up in the Framingham Study. *JAMA*. 1985;254:3449-3453.
19. Brugada R, Tapscott T, Czernuszewicz GZ, et al. Identification of a genetic locus for familial atrial fibrillation. *N Engl J Med*. 1997;336:905-911.
20. Fox CS, Parise H, D'Agostino RB Sr, et al. Parental atrial fibrillation as a risk factor for atrial fibrillation in offspring. *JAMA*. 2004;291:2851-2855.
21. Ellinor PT, Shin JT, Moore RK, et al. Locus for atrial fibrillation maps to chromosome 6q14–16. *Circulation*. 2003;107:2880-2883.
22. Darbar D, Herron KJ, Ballew JD, et al. Familial atrial fibrillation is a genetically heterogeneous disorder. *J Am Coll Cardiol*. 2003;41:2185-2192.

Chapter 3

Classification, diagnosis, and assessment of atrial fibrillation

Atrial fibrillation (AF) can be classified as paroxysmal, persistent, or permanent [1–3] (Figure 3.1). Although such a classification is based on the temporal pattern of the condition and does not reflect the underlying patho-physiological mechanism, it helps in the planning of treatment strategies for the condition.

A first-detected episode of AF is defined as the first episode of AF, regardless of whether or not the patient was symptomatic or the AF self-limited, taking into account the uncertainty about the actual duration of the episode and the possibility of previous undetected episodes [1,2]. AF is considered recurrent when a patient experiences two or more episodes of arrhythmias [1,2]. Recurrent AF may be paroxysmal if it terminates spontaneously, defined by consensus as 7 days. When the AF has been sustained beyond 7 days, it is termed persistent because the arrhythmia requires electrical or pharmacologic

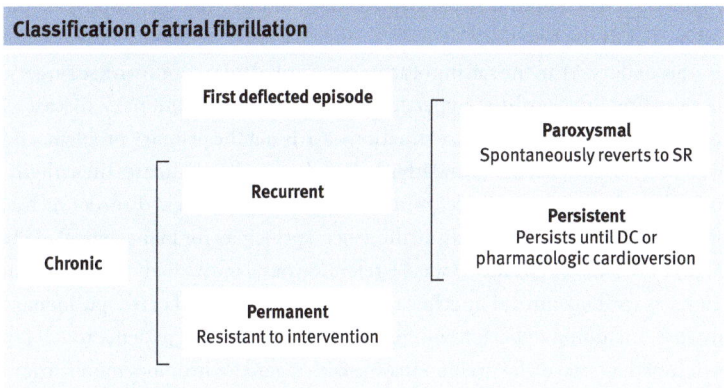

Classification of atrial fibrillation

First deflected episode

Paroxysmal
Spontaneously reverts to SR

Recurrent

Persistent
Persists until DC or pharmacologic cardioversion

Chronic

Permanent
Resistant to intervention

Figure 3.1 Classification of atrial fibrillation. DC, direct current; SR, sinus rhythm.

© Springer Healthcare 2014
Y.G. Yap and A.J. Camm, *Essentials of Atrial Fibrillation*,
DOI 10.1007/978-1-907673-98-6_3

cardioversion for termination. If AF is cardioverted electrically or pharmacologically within 48 hours, it is still termed paroxysmal AF, but if the cardioversion takes place after 48 hours, it is described as persistent. [1,2]. First-detected AF may develop into paroxysmal, persistent, or permanent. AF which lasts over a year, that is not successfully terminated by cardioversion, or when cardioversion has been forgone, is classified as permanent AF [1]. If AF has lasted for more than one year but it is still intended to seek conversion to sinus rhythm, for example by using left atrial ablation, it is known as 'long-standing persistent' AF.

These categories are not mutually exclusive. Paroxysmal AF, in which the frequency of paroxysms is low, may degenerate into either paroxysmal AF with more frequent paroxysms or a sustained form of AF, or the reverse [2]. Similarly, persistent AF may degenerate into permanent AF. In practice, the AF in a given person is categorized by his or her most frequent presentation [2]. The definition of permanent AF is often arbitrary, and the duration refers both to individual episodes and to how long the diagnosis has been present in a given patient. Thus, in a patient with paroxysmal AF, episodes lasting seconds to hours may occur repeatedly for years. This terminology applies to episodes lasting longer than 30 seconds without a reversible cause.

Despite its name, it is possible to revert permanent AF to normal sinus rhythm, especially when the AF is secondary to an underlying treatable cause (eg, hyperthyroidism, pneumonia), or when a specialist procedure such as radiofrequency ablation is performed that modifies the electrophysiologic properties of the heart.

Secondary AF in the setting of acute myocardial infarction, cardiac surgery, pericarditis, myocarditis, hyperthyroidism, or acute pulmonary disease is considered separately. In these situations, AF is not the primary problem, and concurrent treatment of the underlying disorder usually terminates the arrhythmia. Conversely, when AF occurs in the course of a concurrent disorder such as well-controlled hyperthyroidism, the general principles for management of the arrhythmia apply. The term lone AF refers to young individuals aged less than 60 years with no clinical or echocardiographic evidence of cardiopulmonary disease, including hypertension, that may predispose the patients to AF [2]. These patients have a favorable outcome with regard to thromboembolism and mortality. However, over time, patients move out of the lone AF category as a result of aging or development of cardiac abnormalities such as enlargement of the left atrium, and the risks of thromboembolism and mortality may rise [4]. The term non-valvular AF applies to cases with no rheumatic mitral valve disease, prosthetic heart valve, or valve repair [4].

Signs and symptoms

Before treating a patient with AF, it is necessary to consider the patient's symptomatology and the prognostic implications if the arrhythmia is allowed to persist or recur.

AF can present with vague non-specific symptoms or distinct hemodynamic or thromboembolic consequences, or follow an asymptomatic course of unknown duration. Paroxysmal and recurrent AFs are more likely to be symptomatic (Figure 3.2) [5]. When present, symptoms of AF vary with the irregularity and rate of ventricular response, underlying functional status, duration of AF, and individual patient factors [6]. By contrast, patients with permanent AF often have few or no symptoms; this is particularly common in elderly people. Increasingly, silent asymptomatic AF is recognized as an entity and the prevalence is estimated to be around 25–30% [7].

AF can present in the setting of a wide range of cardiac and non-cardiac conditions. The initial diagnosis of AF depends on associating symptoms such as palpitation, dyspnea, dizziness, lightheadedness, syncope, chest pain/discomfort, and fatigue, with the arrhythmia. The symptomatic status of the patient during the arrhythmia should be scored using the EHRA classification [8]. More often than not, AF is detected only after the patient presents with an embolic complication or exacerbation of heart failure. AF associated with a sustained, rapid ventricular response can lead to tachycardia-induced cardiomyopathy. Polyuria may also be present as a result of the release of atrial natriuretic peptide, particularly as episodes of AF start or finish.

The most common presenting symptoms in emergency admissions with newly or previously diagnosed AF are dyspnea, chest pain, and palpitations, with dyspnea being the most common symptom in chronic and recent-onset AF (46.8%), whereas palpitations are the most commonly reported symptom in paroxysmal AF (79.0%) [9–11].

Blood tests

Thyroid function tests are performed to exclude thyrotoxicosis as the cause of AF. Complete blood count and renal function and liver function tests should also be done at baseline in the course of evaluation.

Electrocardiogram

The diagnosis of AF requires electrocardiogram (ECG) documentation during the arrhythmia. An ECG should be performed in all patients, whether or not symptomatic, in whom AF is suspected because an irregular pulse has been detected. Furthermore, the diagnosis of AF requires confirmation by ECG

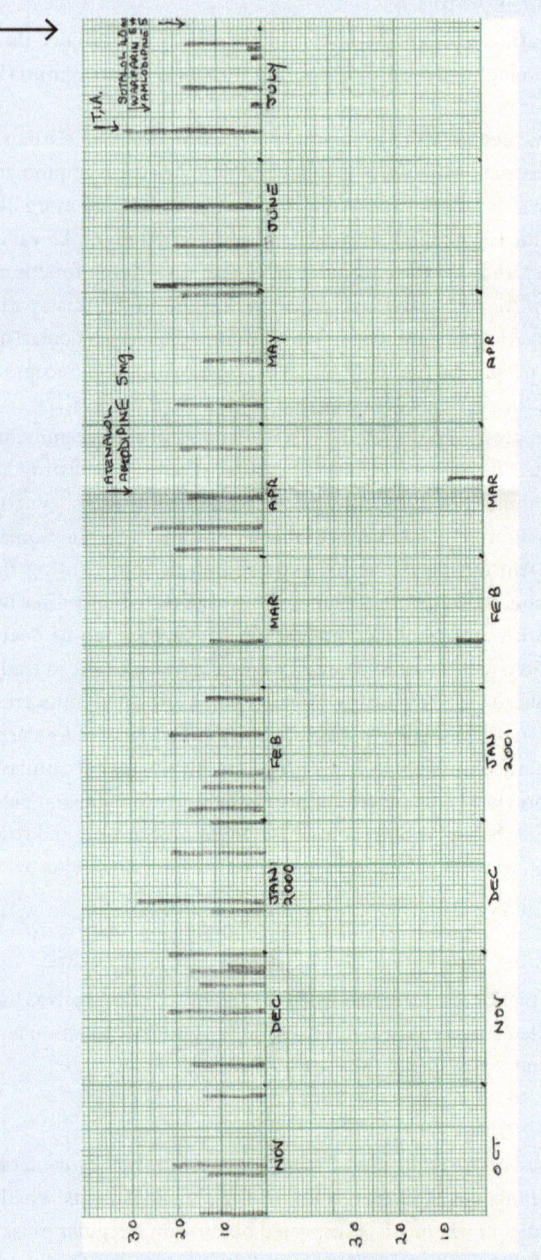

Figure 3.2 A patient's paroxysmal atrial fibrillation diary. The chart is a patient's own paroxysmal AF diary. It shows the patient's record of the frequency (number of vertical bars) and the duration (height of vertical bars) of paroxysmal AF before and after commencing on sotalol treatment. Note that the frequency of AF diminished significantly after the initiation of sotalol treatment (marked ↓).

recording, in the form of either a single-lead rhythm strip, or a 12-lead ECG, bedside telemetry, or ambulatory Holter recordings. A 12-lead ECG can also be used to look for evidence of structural heart disease such as previous infarct, mitral valve disease, and left ventricular hypertrophy.

Many patients with intermittent AF have asymptomatic paroxysms but they remain at risk of complications associated with AF. In patients with daily paroxysms, Holter monitoring for 24 hours may be useful in confirming the diagnosis, but this is less useful in patients who have paroxysms at intervals of more than 24 hours. In the latter group of patients, event ECG recorders (cardiomemos and some implanted loop recorders such as REVEAL [Figure 3.3] and CONFIRM) are commonly used to detect and diagnose AF. Holter monitoring can also be used to assess the rate control in AF and guide drug dosage for rate control or rhythm management. In one study an automatically-triggered event recorder had a higher diagnostic yield than the patient-triggered event recorder, which in turn had a higher diagnostic yield for diagnoses of AF than the 24-hour Holter monitor (24%, 13%, and 5%, respectively, over a 30-day period) [12]. Some patients can also use smart phone ECG recording attachments and applications under the supervision of a medical professional to record, display, store, and transfer single-channel ECG rhythms (Figure 3.4) [13].

Exercise stress testing

Exercise stress testing should be performed if myocardial ischemia is suspected and before initiating type 1C antiarrhythmic drug therapy, which is contraindicated in patients with ischemic heart disease. Furthermore, exercise stress testing can be used to study the adequacy of rate control across a full spectrum of activity, especially during exertion, in patients with persistent or permanent AF.

Chest radiograph

A chest radiograph is useful to detect any intrinsic pulmonary pathology such as pneumonia, bronchial carcinoma, or pulmonary fibrosis, and evaluate the pulmonary vasculature.

Echocardiogram

Transthoracic echocardiography is useful in identifying cardiac abnormalities such as valvular or pericardial disease, atrial enlargement, or left ventricular enlargement, hypertrophy, or dysfunction that predisposes to AF. Similarly, echocardiography has also been used to assess the risk of recurrent AF post-cardioversion, as well as to assess the risk of developing postoperative AF.

Finally, transesophageal echocardiography is often used to guide cardioversion but this is a specialist investigation and requires a skilled cardiologist. Among the transesophageal echocardiography features associated with thromboembolism in patients with non-valvular AF are thrombus, spontaneous echo contrast, reduced left atrial appendage flow velocity (<40 cm/s), and aortic atheromatous abnormalities (Figure 3.5A and B) [14].

Implantable loop recorder and pacemaker log

In about 30% of patients with syncope, the responsible arrhythmic mechanisms remain unrecognized. Implantable loop recorder monitoring facilitates both the identification of mechanisms responsible for recurrent syncope and therapeutic management (Figure 3.3). In patients with implanted pacemakers, defibrillators, or an insertable cardiac monitor, the diagnostic and memory functions of these devices may allow accurate and automatic detection of AF (Figure 3.6).

Medtronic REVEAL® implantable loop recorder

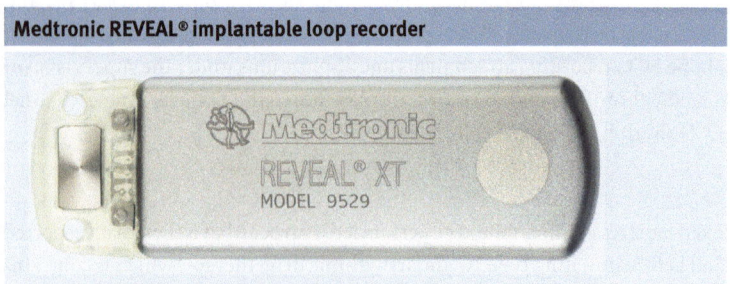

Figure 3.3 Medtronic REVEAL® implantable loop recorder.

AliveCor: an iPhone-based event recorder used for electrocardiograph assessment.

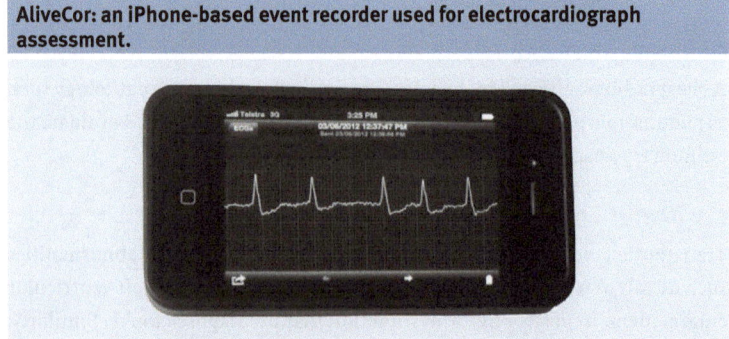

Figure 3.4 AliveCor®: an iPhone-based event recorder used for electrocardiograph assessment.

Transesophageal echocardiography in non-valvular atrial fibrillation

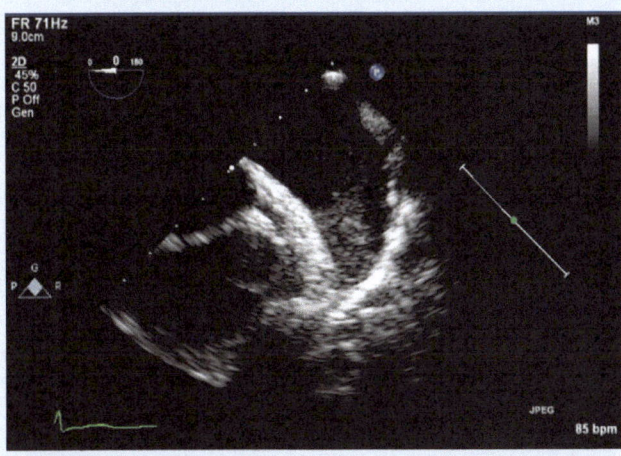

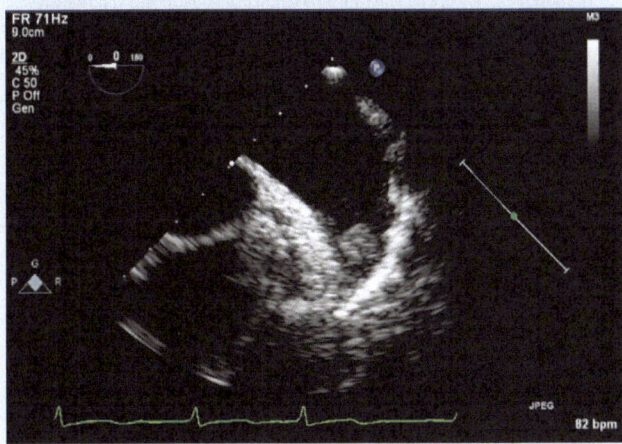

Figure 3.5 A and B Transesophageal echocardiography in non-valvular atrial fibrillation. (A) shows a round thrombus in the left atrial appendage (LAA) of a patient with stroke secondary to persistent atrial fibrillation. **(B)** shows the LAA of the same patient with spontaneous contrast circulating around the LAA thrombus.

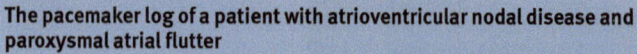

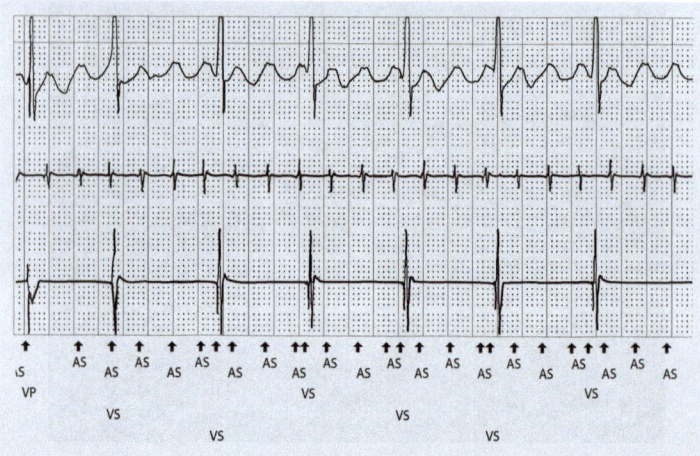

Figure 3.6 The pacemaker log of a patient with atrioventricular nodal disease and paroxysmal atrial flutter. AS, atrial sensing; AV; atrioventricular; VS, ventricular sensing. The patient had a recurrent palpitation and the pacemaker interrogation showed frequent episodes of paroxysmal atrial flutter with 4:1 AV block.

In a study of 34 individuals (60 ± 15 years) with at least two unexplained syncopal episodes and negative neurologic and cardiovascular work-up, during a follow-up of 7 ± 4 months, syncope occurred in 11 individuals [15]. In nine of them, the mechanisms responsible for these events were identified by implantable loop recorder monitoring:
• marked bradycardia or asystole (n = 6);
• AF with wide QRS tachycardia (n = 1); and
• sinus rhythm with fine artifacts likely to be caused by muscle contractions (n = 2).
Presyncope occurred in seven patients: advanced atrioventricular block (n = 3), sinus tachycardia (n = 1), and wide QRS tachycardia (n = 1) were documented. Thus, when considering all 18 patients with recurrent syncope or presyncope, a diagnosis was achieved in 53%. Recognition of the rhythm disorder in seven patients with syncope and four patients with presyncope helped guide patient management [15].

With the technology of an implantable loop recorder, it is feasible to characterize the ECG events preceding AF onset, which typically demonstrate a varied pattern within individuals. However, there is significant incongruity between symptoms and ECG AF burden [16]. Thus, an insertable cardiac monitor is recommended for accurate characterization of AF burden [16].

In another study of patients with unexplained syncope, structural heart disease, and negative electrophysiologic study, the implantation of a loop recorder revealed that the mechanism of syncope was heterogeneous [17]. During a follow-up of 3–15 months in this study of 35 patients, syncope recurred in 6 (17%); in 3 patients, the mechanism of syncope was bradycardia with long pauses (sudden-onset atrioventricular block in 2 cases and sinus arrest in 1); in 1 patient, there was stable sinus tachycardia, and in 2 patients, who had chronic AF, there was an increase in ventricular rate [17]. A total of 23 episodes of presyncope were documented in 8 patients (23%):

- no rhythm variation or mild tachycardia in 12 cases;
- paroxysmal AF or atrial tachycardia in 10 cases; and
- sustained ventricular tachycardia in 1 case.

References

1. Gallagher MM, Camm AJ. Classification of atrial fibrillation. *PACE*. 1997;20:1603-1605.
2. Fuster V, Rydén LE, Cannom DS, American College of Cardiology Foundation/American Heart Association Task Force, et al. 2011 ACCF/AHA/HRS focused updates incorporated into the ACC/AHA/ESC 2006 guidelines for the management of patients with atrial fibrillation: a report of the American College of Cardiology Foundation/American Heart Association Task Force on practice guidelines. *Circulation*. 2011;123:e269-e367.
3. National Collaborating Centre for Chronic Conditions. Atrial Fibrillation: National guideline for management in primary and secondary care. London: Royal College of Physicians;2006.
4. Kopecky SL, Gersh BJ, McGoon MD, et al. The natural history of lone atrial fibrillation. A population-based study over three decades. *N Engl J Med*. 1987;317:669-674.
5. Saveliea I, Camm AJ. Atrial fibrillation – all change. *Clin Med*. 2007;7: 374-379.
6. Kerr CR, Boone J, Connolly SJ, et al. The Canadian Registry of Atrial Fibrillation: a noninterventional follow-up of patients after the first diagnosis of atrial fibrillation. *Am J Cardiol*. 1998;82:82-5N.
7. Saveliea I, Camm AJ. Clinical relevance of silent atrial fibrillation: prevalence, prognosis, quality of life, and management. *J Interv Card Electrophysiol*. 2000;4:369-382.
8. European Heart Rhythm Association; European Association for Cardio-Thoracic Surgery; Camm AJ, Kirchhof P, Lip GY, et al. Guidelines for the management of atrial fibrillation: the Task Force for the Management of Atrial Fibrillation of the European Society of Cardiology (ESC). *Eur Heart J*. 2010;19:2369-2429,
9. Zarifis J, Beevers G, Lip GY. Acute admissions with atrial fibrillation in a British multiracial hospital population. *Br J Clin Pract*.1997;51:91-96.
10. Burton JH, Vinson DR, Drummond K, et al. Electrical cardioversion of emergency department patients with atrial fibrillation. *Ann Emerg Med*. 2004;44:20-30.
11. van Walraven C, Hart RG, Wells GA, et al. A clinical prediction rule to identify patients with atrial fibrillation and a low risk for stroke while taking aspirin. *Arch Intern Med*. 2003;163:936-943.
12. Reiffel JA, Schwarzberg R, Murry M. Comparison of autotriggered memory loop recorders versus standard loop recorders versus 24-hour Holter monitors for arrhythmia detection. *Am J Cardiol*. 2005;95:1055-1059.

13. Lau J, Lowres N, Neubeck L, et al. Abstract 16810: Validation of an iPhone ECG application suitable for community screening for silent atrial fibrillation: a novel way to prevent stroke. *Circulation*. 2012;126:A16810.

14. Zabalgoitia M, Halperin JL, Pearce LA, et al. Transesophageal echocardiographic correlates of clinical risk of thromboembolism in nonvalvular atrial fibrillation. Stroke Prevention in Atrial Fibrillation III Investigators. *J Am Coll Cardiol*. 1998;31:1622-1626.

15. Lombardi F, Calosso E, Mascioli G, et al. Utility of implantable loop recorder (Reveal Plus) in the diagnosis of unexplained syncope. *Europace*. 2005;7:19-24.

16. Schwartzman D, Blagev DP, Brown ML, Mehra R. Electrocardiographic events preceding onset of atrial fibrillation: insights gained using an implantable loop recorder. *J Cardiovasc Electrophysiol*. 2006;17:243-246.

17. Menozzi C, Brignole M, Garcia-Civera R, et al; International Study on Syncope of Uncertain Etiology (ISSUE) Investigators. Mechanism of syncope in patients with heart disease and negative electrophysiologic test. *Circulation*. 2002;105:2741-2745.

Chapter 4

Rate and rhythm control strategies for atrial fibrillation

Rate control versus rhythm control

Before treating a patient with atrial fibrillation (AF), it is necessary to consider the patient's symptomatology and the prognostic implications if the arrhythmia were allowed to persist or recur. Essentially, the treatment for AF can be divided into two main treatment strategies: rate control and rhythm control [1]. For rate control, the use of chronotropic drugs or electrophysiologic ablation is required to reduce the rapid ventricular rate often found in patients with AF (unless the patient has concurrent atrioventricular block). Although the atria continue to fibrillate with this strategy, it improves the symptoms and reduces the risk of associated morbidity such as tachycardia-induced cardiomyopathy. The risk of thromboembolism remains as a result of the persistence of the AF; however, this risk may be reduced by administering antithrombotic drugs.

Rate control strategy for atrial fibrillation

When a relapse occurs in patients with paroxysmal AF, it is important to control the ventricular rate if the patients are symptomatic or hemodynamically compromised by it. In patients with permanent AF, rate control is also necessary to improve the quality of life and distressing symptoms, and prevent left ventricular dysfunction. Generally, a target resting heart rate <80 beats/min at rest and <115 beats/min during light and moderate exercise is aimed for [2]. There are three classes of drugs to choose from for rate control:

- digitalis;
- β-blockers; and
- calcium channel blockers.

© Springer Healthcare 2014
Y.G. Yap and A.J. Camm, *Essentials of Atrial Fibrillation*,
DOI 10.1007/978-1-907673-98-6_4

The American Heart Association/American College of Cardiology/European Society of Cardiology (ESC) guidelines suggested that β-blockers or the calcium channel blockers diltiazem and verapamil should be used in most patients with chronic AF without heart failure, whereas in patients with heart failure, digoxin or even the antiarrhythmic amiodarone should be used to control heart rate [3,4]. Intravenous amiodarone is not effectivefor acute conversion (<1 hour) but may still be useful for late conversion and is successful in over 80% of cases within 24 hours [2]. Digoxin provides rate control during rest but its effect is not maintained during exercise, so it is very useful in elderly people with a low level of activity. The dose should be titrated against resting heart rate [2]. Several studies have tried to establish whether lenient rate control (eg, <110 beats per minute at rest) or strict rate control (eg, <80 beats/min at rest and <110 beats/min during moderate exercise) is preferable. Strict rate control is only advised when lenient control leaves the patient with symptoms due to the arrhythmia.

When rapid control of the ventricular response to AF is required or oral administration of medication is not feasible, intravenous medication such as diltiazem may be considered [6]. Otherwise, in hemodynamically stable patients with a rapid ventricular response to AF, negative chronotropic medication may be administered orally. Combinations may be necessary to achieve rate control in both acute and chronic situations. Some patients may develop symptomatic bradycardia that requires permanent pacing.

For acute rate control of AF in patients without heart failure or accessory pathway, intravenous β-blockers (esmolol, metoprolol, and propranolol), diltiazem, or verapamil may be used as first-line treatment. For patients with heart failure with no accessory pathway, intravenous digoxin or amiodarone may be used to control the heart rate of AF. Among patients with AF and accessory pathway, only intravenous amiodarone is indicated for use [2]. Intravenous β-blockers need to be used with caution for fear of unsuspected heart failure due to their negative inotropic effects, except in AF associated with thyrotoxicosis where β-blockers are preferred [3].

Rhythm control strategy for atrial fibrillation

For rhythm control, the use of cardioversion is required to convert AF to normal sinus rhythm. There are two types of cardioversion: electrical and pharmacologic. However, not all attempts at cardioversion are successful. At 1 year after cardioversion, approximately 50% of patients revert back into AF [6].

In patients presenting with acute-onset AF within 48 hours, pharmacologic cardioversion is the preferred strategy, whereas electrical cardioversion is the standard procedure where the AF is more prolonged. Cardioversion is not normally attempted until possible underlying precipitants (eg, thyrotoxicosis, infections) have been successfully treated and any electrolyte abnormalities corrected. Younger patients with normal hearts who develop AF after an alcohol binge do not require cardioversion because these cases usually revert back to sinus rhythm spontaneously.

Patients may be prescribed antiarrhythmic drugs before and/or after successful electrical cardioversion for a period of time, or even long term to help prevent recurrent AF. The rhythm control strategies may also require the appropriate administration of antithrombotic therapy to reduce the risk of thromboembolic events, depending on the type of AF [3,4]. There is no evidence that the risk of thromboembolism or stroke differs between pharmacologic and electrical methods of cardioversion. The recommendations for anticoagulation are therefore the same for both methods. Anticoagulation (INR 2.0–3.0) is recommended for 3 weeks before and at least 4 weeks after cardioversion for patients with AF of unknown duration or with AF >48 hours [5,7]. Patients with cardiac failure, hypertension, age ≥75 (doubled), diabetes, stroke (doubled)-vascular disease, age 65–74 and sex category (female) (CHA_2DS_2-VASc) risk above or equal to 1 require ongoing thromboemboltic propylaxis with warfarin.

A 2012 update to the ESC guidelines also recommends intravenous flecainide, propafenone, ibulitide, or vernakalent in patients without heart failure, and gives a cautious recommendation to intravenous vernakalent for patients with moderate structural heart failure (but not those with New York Heart Association [NYHA] class I-II heart failure) [5].

Direct current cardioversion

All patients with persistent AF should be considered for cardioversion by drugs or direct current (DC) shock regardless of symptoms, unless there are contraindications to cardioversion. Cardioversion is indicated only in patients with paroxysmal AF if, as often occurs eventually, it becomes persistent and efforts are going to be made to maintain sinus rhythm after cardioversion. Before cardioversion, it is important to assess each patient individually for its appropriateness as well as the probability of successful cardioversion and the likelihood of maintaining sinus rhythm thereafter. The indication of cardioversion is generally based on clinical setting. Several factors can affect the success of the cardioversion and recurrence of AF:

- age of patient;
- rheumatic mitral valve disease;
- duration of arrhythmia;
- left atrial size;
- functional class; and

• possibly concomitant administration of antiarrhythmic drugs.

Patients aged >50 years and with underlying rheumatic mitral valve disease are associated with poor success rate of cardioversion [8,9], whereas prolonged AF duration (>1 year), large atrial size (>55 mm), rheumatic mitral valve disease, and low functional class (≥NYHA III) [10–12] are associated with recurrence of AF. These factors are mostly applied to DC cardioversion but the same factors probably also influence the results of pharmacologic cardioversion.

DC cardioversion has been successfully used to restore sinus rhythm in approximately 90% of patients with chronic AF (Figure 4.1) [13]. All patients undergoing electrical cardioversion will require oral anticoagulation for 3 weeks before the procedure and for 4 weeks afterwards [14–16]. In new-onset AF, it is generally thought to be safe to cardiovert without anticoagulation if the cardioversion is undertaken within 48 hours of its onset [2]. However, in practice, intravenous heparin is generally given immediately on diagnosis while the decision regarding the appropriateness of DC cardioversion and the preparation for the procedure are being carried out. This is then followed by 4 weeks of oral anticoagulant therapy. If the patient has a dilated left atrium or mitral valve disease, formal oral anticoagulant treatment for 3 weeks is necessary before DC cardioversion, even if the onset is within 48 hours.

There has been extensive experience with vitamin K antagonists (VKAs) as anticoagulant therapy for cardioversion, but more recently dabigatran, and other novel oral anticoagulants have been used in a similar manner to VKAs.

DC cardioversion is performed under heavy sedation or short-acting general anesthetics (eg, intravenous propofol) and the usual general anesthetic assessment should be carried out before the procedure. Hypokalemia and supratherapeutic levels of digoxin can precipitate ventricular arrhythmias with DC cardioversion, so their levels should be checked before the procedure. The skin is covered with a gel pad. The paddles can be placed in either

Successful external DC cardioversion

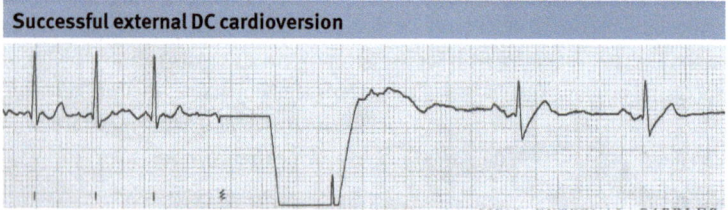

Figure 4.1 Successful external DC cardioversion. The figure shows the emergence of sinus rhythm after the cardioversion artifact. For standard monophasic cardioversion, an initial energy of 200J (monophasic) or 150J (biphasic) is usually required, building up to 360J or 200J, respectively, J if necessary. Synchronization is used to avoid discharging on the T wave, resulting in ventricular arrhythmias.

anteroanterior position (right 2nd interspace versus apex) or anteroposterior position (left precordial against left subscapular), although there is controversy about the optimal paddle position for DC cardioversion. Synchronization is used to avoid discharging on the T wave, resulting in ventricular arrhythmias. For monophasic DC cardioversion, an initial 300 J biphasic shock or 150J monophasic shock should then be given. If this fails to restore sinus rhythm, a second shock of 300J biphasic (or 200 J monophasic) can be delivered. If this also fails to cardiovert, a third and final shock of similar magnitude can then be given. Biphasic shocks at high output are more successful than equivilant monophasic waveforms. Cardioversion should be abandoned if it is unsuccessful after the third shock. A second attempt at cardioversion should be tried, with the antiarrhythmic drug changed to amiodarone for 6 weeks, if the patient is not already on the treatment. It is prudent that patients undergoing DC cardioversion for AF are on some kind of antiarrhythmic. This is to improve the probability of successful cardioversion, demonstrated by amiodarone and esmolol [17,18], or to maintain sinus rhythm after successful cardioversion. Figure 4.2 shows the Vaughan-Williams classifica-

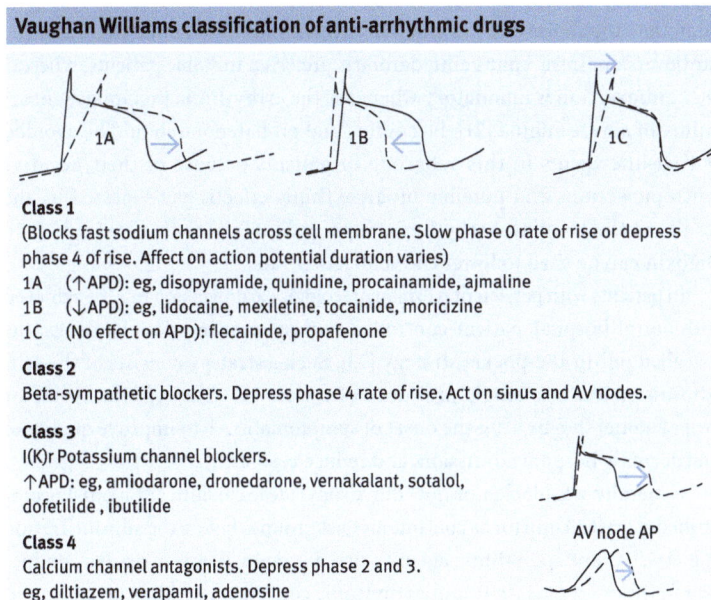

Vaughan Williams classification of anti-arrhythmic drugs

Class 1
(Blocks fast sodium channels across cell membrane. Slow phase 0 rate of rise or depress phase 4 of rise. Affect on action potential duration varies)
1A ($\uparrow$APD): eg, disopyramide, quinidine, procainamide, ajmaline
1B ($\downarrow$APD): eg, lidocaine, mexiletine, tocainide, moricizine
1C (No effect on APD): flecainide, propafenone

Class 2
Beta-sympathetic blockers. Depress phase 4 rate of rise. Act on sinus and AV nodes.

Class 3
I(K)r Potassium channel blockers.
$\uparrow$APD: eg, amiodarone, dronedarone, vernakalant, sotalol, dofetilide , ibutilide

Class 4
Calcium channel antagonists. Depress phase 2 and 3.
eg, diltiazem, verapamil, adenosine

AV node AP

Figure 4.2 Vaughan-Williams classification of antiarrhythmic drugs. AP, action potential; APD, action potential duration; AV, atrioventricular.

tion of antiarrhythmic drugs. After successful DC cardioversion, it may take at least 3 weeks for full atrial mechanical activity to be restored [15]. It is therefore important that both antiarrhythmic and anticoagulant therapy are continued for at least this period of time. Most of the antiarrhythmic benefit post cardioversion is achieved by continuing the therapy for about 4 weeks.

For acute pharmacologic cardioversion, oral or intravenous administration of class Ic (flecainide and propafenone) or III (amiodarone, ibutilide, dofetilide) antiarrhythmic drugs, or the atrial selective agent vernakalant, can be used [19]. The conversion rate for flecainide ranges between 59% and 93% for the intravenous route and between 56% and 81% for the oral route. Most of the conversions are achieved within the first hour. The success rate for propafenone ranges between 42% and 88% when given intravenously and between 50% and 81% for the oral route [20]. The conversion is usually achieved in the first hour for the intravenous route and between 2 and 3 hours for the oral route. These drugs should therefore be used as first choice for conversion of acute paroxysm of AF.

It is important to note that, in patients with AF after acute myocardial infarction, the choice of treatment is between intravenous amiodarone and DC cardioversion. Intravenous amiodarone is preferred in stable patients, whereas DC cardioversion is mandatory whenever the arrhythmia precipitates heart failure or severe angina [21]. Flecainide and propafenone should be avoided as first-line agents in this subgroup of patients because of their negative inotropic actions and possible proarrhythmic effects, as suggested by the results of the Cardiac Arrhythmia Suppression Trial with flecainide [22]. Digoxin can be used to lower the ventricular rate.

In patients with persistent AF, pharmacologic cardioversion may be achieved with out-of-hospital, patient-controlled conversion using class 1C drugs, the so-called pill-in-the-pocket strategy [23]. Such a strategy consists of the self-administration of a single oral dose of a class 1C drug (eg, flecainide or propafenone) shortly after the onset of symptomatic AF to improve quality of life, decrease hospital admission, and reduce cost [4,23].

Generally, a β-blocker or non-dihydropyridine calcium antagonist is prescribed at least 30 min (or as continuous background) before the administration of a class 1C antiarrhythmic agent to prevent rapid atrioventricular conduction in the event of class 1C antiarrhythmic conversion of AF to atrial flutter. Furthermore, an initial conversion trial should be carried out in hospital in case of bradycardia after termination of paroxysmal AF due to sinus node or atrioventricular node dysfunction [4].

Maintenance of sinus rhythm

Maintenance of sinus rhythm is just as important a treatment strategy as restoration of sinus rhythm in patients with paroxysmal or persistent AF to prevent recurrences. European clinical guidelines recommend that flecainide, propafenone, sotalol, or dronedarone are first-line agents in patients with lone atrial fibrillation or minimal structural heart disease. Amiodarone is reserved for patients with congestive heart failure or significant left ventricular hypertrophy, or as a second-line agent after failure of other antiarrhythmic drugs, because of its potential serious extra-cardiac side-effects [4]. In a multicenter, double-blind, crossover study, Anderson et al. showed that flecainide prolonged the median time to the first recurrence (15 vs 3 days, $P<0.001$) and the time interval between subsequent attacks from 6 days to 27 days compared with placebo ($P<0.001$) [21]. Other workers also reported flecainide to be effective in long-term suppression of paroxysmal AF in between 49% and 73% of patients [24,25], even in those previously resistant to quinidine therapy. Propafenone is also effective in maintaining sinus rhythm in 40% of patients with drug-refractory or chronic AF after successful DC cardioversion [26]. Dronedarone is pharmacologically related to amiodarone but has a reduced risk of side effects. As a consequence of the PALLAS trial, the European Medicines Agency stated that patients with permanent AF should not be treated with dronedarone, particularly those with a significant cardiovascular disease burden. The drug can still be used in patients with paroxysmal or persistent AF after cardioversion provided that there is no history of significant heart failure [27].

Amiodarone is effective in maintaining sinus rhythm in 53–97% of patients with chronic and paroxysmal AF, and it is especially useful in patients refractory to other drugs [27–32]. In contrast to class 1C drugs, amiodarone is associated with a lower proarrhythmic risk and is safe for long-term use, particularly in patients after an acute myocardial infarction or with left ventricular dysfunction [33]. However, it is important to be aware that long-term amiodarone use has a relatively high incidence of extracardiac side effects, particularly hyper- or hypothyroidism, corneal deposits, peripheral neuropathy, abnormal liver enzymes, and pulmonary fibrosis [33,34]. The current choice of antiarrhythmic drugs related to underlying pathophysiology is summarized in Figure 4.3 [5].

Treatment strategy for paroxysmal atrial fibrillation

The aim of treatment for paroxysmal AF [1] is to:

• suppress the paroxysms of AF;

• maintain long-term sinus rhythm; and

• prevent thromboembolic complications associated with paroxysmal AF.

Choice of antiarrhythmic drug according to underlying pathology

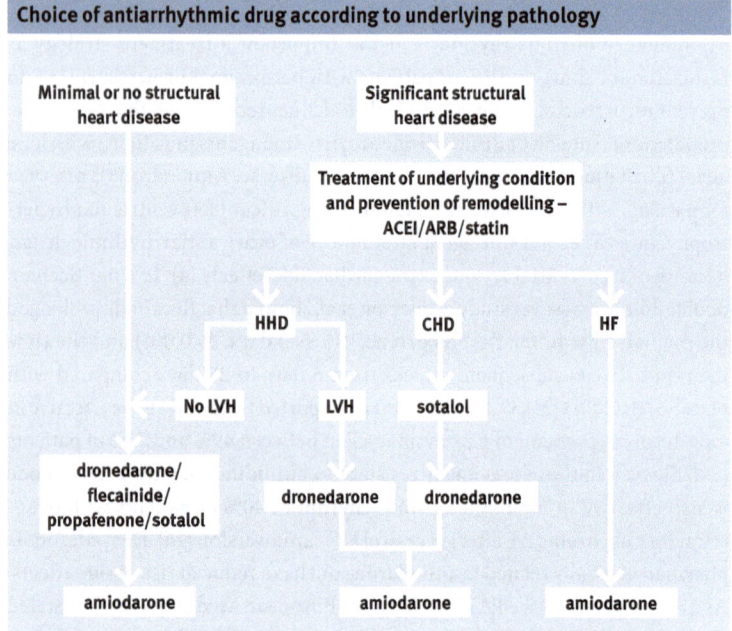

Figure 4.3 Choice of antiarrhythmic drug according to underlying pathology. ACEI, angiotensin-converting enzyme inhibitor; ARB, angiotensin-receptor blocker; HHD, hypertensive heart disease; CHD, coronary heart disease; HF, heart failure; LVH, left ventricular hypertrophy, NYHA, New York Heart Association. Reproduced with permission from Camm et al [5].

In practice, few patients achieve complete suppression of paroxysms of AF. Patients with paroxysmal AF should be advised to avoid precipitating factors such as caffeine, alcohol, and stress, and recieve adequate treatment of underlying diseases such as myocardial ischemia, thyrotoxicosis, and heart failure [35]. If episodes of paroxysmal AF are infrequent or symptoms are induced by known precipitants as mentioned above, a no drug treatment strategy or a pill-in-the-pocket approach may be considered for longer lasting paroxyms, provided that the patient does not have any history of left ventricular dysfunction or valvular or ischemic heart disease [1].

In patients with symptomatic paroxysms (with or without structural heart disease or coronary artery disease), a standard β-blocker should be the initial treatment option. For patients with paroxysmal AF and no structural heart disease, where symptomatic suppression is not achieved with standard β-blockers, either a class 1C agent (such as flecainide or propafenone), sotalol (with gradual titration) or dronedarone should be given. If these pharmaco-logic treatments have been unsuccessful in suppressing the paroxysms, either amiodarone or non-pharmacologic intervention should be considered [1].

In patients with paroxysmal AF with poor left ventricular function, where symptoms are adequately suppressed by standard β-blockers given as part of the routine heart failure management strategy, no further treatment for par-oxysms is needed. However, if standard β-blockers do not adequately suppress paroxysms, amiodarone should be tried and if it is unsuccessful, referral for non-pharmacologic intervention should be considered [1].

It is essential that patients have their symptoms and medication reviewed regularly to assess for any side effects of medications, the need for continuing treatment, and the need to reduce the dosage of medications.

Treatment strategies for persistent atrial fibrillation

The treatment strategies for persistent AF with either rate control or rhythm control should not be mutually exclusive. The potential advantages and disad-vantages of each strategy, and any indications that might favor one approach rather than the other, should be explained to patients before agreeing which to adopt. For both strategies, appropriate antithrombotic therapy should be used [1] (see Chapter 5). No antiarrhythmic drug is required to maintain sinus rhythm in patients with persistent AF as a result of reversible causes, and cardioversion can be successfully performed provided that there are no risk factors for recurrence.

A rate-control strategy should be the preferred initial option in the following patients with persistent AF [1]:
- age >65 years;
- with coronary artery disease;
- with contraindications to antiarrhythmic drugs;
- unsuitable for cardioversion, including those with:
  - contraindications to anticoagulation, structural heart disease (eg, large left atrium > 5.5 cm, mitral stenosis) that precludes long-term maintenance of sinus rhythm
  - a long duration of AF (usually >12 months)
  - history of multiple failed attempts at cardioversion and/or relapses, even with concomitant use of antiarrhythmic drugs or non-pharmacologic approaches
  - an ongoing but reversible cause of AF (eg, thyrotoxicosis); and
- without congestive heart failure.

A rhythm-control strategy should be the preferred initial option in the following patients with persistent AF [1]:

- with symptomatic disease;
- younger patients;
- presenting for the first time with lone AF;
- with AF secondary to a treated/corrected precipitant; and
- with congestive heart failure.

However, in patients with persistent AF who require antiarrhythmic drugs to maintain sinus rhythm and who have structural heart disease (coronary artery disease or left ventricular dysfunction), a standard β-blocker should be the first-line treatment, with amiodarone being the second option. For those patients without structural heart disease, a β-blocker should still be the initial treatment option with a class 1C agent, dronedarone or sotalol as the second-line treatment and amiodarone as the final option if other drugs are ineffective, contraindicated, or not tolerated [3].

Treatment strategy for permanent atrial fibrillation

The objective of treatment in permanent AF is to minimize the symptoms associated with excessive tachycardia and to prevent tachycardia-induced cardiomyopathy [35]. It has been suggested that, for optimal rate control, the resting heart rate should be <80 beats/min and peak exercise heart rate <(220−age) beats/min [36].

For rate control in patients with permanent AF, β-blockers or rate-limiting non-dihydropyridine calcium antagonists (diltiazem and verapamil) should be the preferred initial monotherapy in all patients. Digoxin should be considered as monotherapy only in predominately sedentary patients.

In patients with permanent AF where monotherapy is inadequate, β-blockers or rate-limiting calcium antagonists should be given with digoxin to control the heart rate during normal activities. However, to control the heart rate during both normal activities and exercise, rate-limiting calcium antagonists should be given with digoxin [1].

Surgical ablation

The surgical Maze procedure involves incising and sewing the atria into complex pieces at critical locations to create barriers to conduction and prevent sustained AF. The procedure creates transmural lesions to isolate the pulmonary veins (PV) and prevent PV tachycardia from conducting into the atrium, and connects these dividing lines to the mitral valve annulus, thus creating electrical barriers in the left atrium that prevent sustained macroentrant rhythms [37].

Over the years, changes in techniques of the classic maze were made, culminating in the cut-and-sew Cox–Maze III procedure, which incorporates four lesion sets as the gold standard:

1. encirclement of the PVs;
2. a lesion joining the circumferential PV lesion to the mitral annulus, with amputation of the left atrial appendage;
3. a circumferential lesion in the coronary sinus; and
4. ablation of the right atrium.

The success rates of surgical Maze procedures vary from 70% to 95% at the 15-year follow-up [38,39]. When combined with resection of the left atrial appendage, postoperative thromboembolic events are substantially reduced. The risks of surgical Maze ablation include death (<1%), need for permanent pacing, recurrent bleeding requiring reoperation, impaired atrial transport function, delayed atrial arrhythmias (especially atrial flutter), and atrioesophageal fistula [40]. Despite its high success rate, the Maze operation has not been widely adopted other than for patients undergoing cardiac surgery as a result of the need for cardiopulmonary bypass. New surgical approaches for AF therapy utilize radiofrequency or other sources for an easy ablation during open-heart surgery. However, freedom from AF has still been found to be superior after standard Maze III compared with radiofrequency modifications, both soon after the operation and later. Patients undergoing radiofrequency ablation are 4.5 times more likely to be in AF at discharge (95% CI 1.8–10.9) and 5 times more likely to be in AF at follow-up (95% CI 1.4–17.3) [41,42].

However, recent advances in the development of new ablation technologies allow surgeons to perform PV ablation, create linear left atrial lesions, and remove the left atrial appendage rapidly and safely [43]. Lesions are created under direct vision, minimizing the risk of damage to the PVs and adjacent mediastinal structures. Most surgical ablation procedures have been performed together with mitral valve surgery, with the combination of mitral valve repair, resection of left atrial appendage, and cure of AF enabling patients to avoid long-term anticoagulation [43]. More recently developed surgical instrumentation now enables keyhole thoracoscopic approaches, facilitating extension of epicardial catheter-based AF ablation and excision of the left atrial appendage, on patients with isolated AF and no other indication for cardiac surgery. In addition, investigational novel devices, designed specifically for minimally invasive epicardial exclusion of the left atrial appendage, will broaden the range of treatment options for patients with AF, possibly eliminating the need for anticoagulation in selected patients [43]. This minimally invasive thoracoscopic approach can be performed off pump, thus avoiding a median sternotomy, cardiopulmonary bypass, and cardioplegic arrest perioperatively, and ensuring a shorter, less painful recovery. If the efficacy of these adaptations approaches that of the endocardial Maze procedure and they can be performed safely, they may become acceptable alternatives for a larger proportion of patients with AF.

Catheter ablation for atrial fibrillation

Catheter ablation of AF is now a realistic therapeutic option across a broad spectrum of patients [44]. The following are patients who may be considered for catheter ablation:

- patients with symptomatic paroxysmal AF who have failed at least one antiarrhythmic drug;
- patients with long-lasting, symptomatic, persistent AF who have failed treatment with more than one conventional antiarrhythmic drug, electrical cardioversion, or both.

In almost half of patients with long-lasting persistent AF, a second procedure is necessary to maintain sinus rhythm, and there are no absolute exclusion criteria or a predetermined limit to the number of procedures performed per patient.

Patients with both AF and moderate-to-severe left ventricular impairment may also be considered for catheter ablation [45,46]. Currently, this is limited to patients with AF, echocardiographic evidence of left ventricular dysfunction, heart failure symptoms of NYHA class II or more, and the absence of an alternative explanation for their cardiac dysfunction [47].

The concept of catheter-based AF ablation arises from the observation that AF could be triggered from ectopics originating from the ostia of the PVs, and the demonstration that elimination of these foci abolished AF. Initially, areas of automaticity and/or local re-entry within the PVs were targeted, but subsequent research demonstrated that potentials may arise in multiple regions of the right and left atria, and modification of the procedures has incorporated linear left atrial ablation, mitral isthmus ablation, or both for selected patients [48]. The technique of ablation has continued to evolve and encompasses the following:

- circumferential electrical isolation of the entire PV musculature;
- use of a non-fluoroscopic guidance system;
- radiofrequency energy delivered circumferentially outside the ostia of the PV; and
- radiofrequency catheter ablation targeting complex fractionated electrograms [4].

The stepwise approach in which several strategies are combined (pulmonary vein isolation, targeting of fractionated potentials, and linear lesions), suggesting that all the targets contributed to the maintenance of AF, has resulted in unprecedented success in maintaining sinus rhythm in the medium term, with recovery of atrial mechanical function in patients with long-lasting persistent AF [47]. With this approach, termination of AF occurred in 87% of cases [49], resulting in freedom from sinus rhythm at 1 year in 95% of patients [50]. A more recent technique involves identification and ablation of anchor points of left atrial spiral waves.

Despite these advances, the long-term efficacy of catheter ablation in the treatment of AF remains unclear, especially since patients can have recurrent AF without symptoms. Therefore, it remains uncertain whether apparent cures represent elimination of AF or transformation into an asymptomatic form of paroxysmal AF. Major complications of catheter ablation for AF have been reported in about 5% or 6% of procedures and include PV stenosis, thromboembolism (including embolic stroke, atrio-esophageal fistula, and left atrial flutter), cardiac tamponade, PV occlusion with hemoptysis, and vascular injury requiring surgical repair and/or transfusion [51,52].

References

1. National Collaborating Centre for Chronic Conditions. Atrial Fibrillation: National clinical Guideline for Management in Primary and Secondary Care. London: Royal College of Physicians;2006:49.
2. Crijns HJGM, Van Gelder IC, Tieleman RG, Van Gilst WH. Atrial fibrillation: antiarrhythmic therapy. In: Yusuf S, Cairns JA, Camm AJ, Fallen EL, Gersh BJ (eds), *Evidence Based Cardiology*. London: BMJ Books;1998: 527-543.
3. Gallagher MM, Kishore AGR, Camm AJ. Management Strategies in atrial fibrillation. In: McEwan JR (ed.), *Current Issues in Cardiology. Management strategies*. London: BMJ Publishing Group;1998: 185-225.
4. Fuster V, Rydén LE, Cannom DS, et al. 2011 ACCF/AHA/HRS focused updates incorporated into the ACC/AHA/ESC 2006 Guidelines for the management of patients with atrial fibrillation: a report of the American College of Cardiology Foundation/American Heart Association Task Force on Practice Guidelines. *Circulation*. 2011;123:e269-e367.
5. Camm AJ, Yip GYH, De Caterina R, et al. 2012 focused update of the ESC Guidelines for the management of atrial fibrillation: an update of the 2010 ESC Guidelines for the management of atrial fibrillation. Developed with the special contribution of the European Heart Rhythm Association. *Eur Heart J*. 2012;33:2719-2747.
6. Lim H, Hamaad A, Lip G. Clinical review: clinical management of atrial fibrillation – rate control versus rhythm control. *Crit Care*. 2004;8:271-279.
7. Gallagher MM, Guo X-H, Poloniecki JD, et al. Initial energy setting, outcome and efficiency in direct current cardioversion of atrial fibrillation and flutter. *J Am Coll Cardiol*. 2001;38:1498-1504.
8. Brodsky MA, Allen BJ, Capparelli EV, et al. Factors determining maintenance of sinus rhythm after cardioversion in chronic atrial fibrillation with left atrial dilatation. *Am J Cardiol*. 1989;63:1065-1068.

9. Waris E, Kreus KE, Salokannel J. Factors influencing persistence of sinus rhythm after DC shock treatment of atrial fibrillation. *Acta Med Scand*. 1971;189:161–166.
10. Szekeley P, Sideris D, Batson G. Maintenance of sinus rhythm after atrial fibrillation. *Br Heart J*. 1970;32:741-746.
11. Van Gelder IC, Crijns HJGM, Tieleman RG et al. Value and limitation of electrical cardioversion in patients with chronic atrial fibrillation – importance of arrhythmia risk factors and oral anticoagulation. *Arch Intern Med*. 1996;156:2585-2592.
12. Crijns HJGM, Gosselink ATM, Van Gelder IC et al. Drugs after cardioversion to prevent relapses of chronic atrial fibrillation. In: Kingma JH, van Hemel NM, Lie KI (eds), *Atrial Fibrillation, A Treatable Disease?* Dordrecht: Kluwer Academic Publishers, 1992:105-148.
13. Lown B, Amarasingham R, Neuman J. New method for terminating cardiac arrhythmias. *JAMA*. 1962;182:548-555.
14. Laupacis A, Albers G, Dalend J, et al. Antithrombotic therapy in atrial fibrillation. *Chest*. 1995;108:3528-3595.
15. Manning WJ, Leeman DE, Gotch PJ, et al. Pulsed Doppler evaluation of atrial mechanical function after electrical cardioversion of atrial fibrillation. *J Am Coll Cardiol*. 1989;13:617-623.
16. Padraig GO, Puleo PR, Bolli R, et al. Return of atrial mechanical function following electrical cardioversion of atrial dysrhythmia. *Am Heart J*. 1990;120:353-359.
17. Newby KH, Waugh R, Hardee M, et al. Amiodarone decreases defibrillation threshold in patients undergoing elective cardioversion for atrial fibrillation (abstr). *Circulation*. 1996;94:I-667.
18. Niebauer M, Chung MK, Holmes D, et al. Esmolol reduces atrial defibrillation thresholds: a randomized, placebo-controlled study. *J Am Coll Cardiol*. 1997;29:292A.
19. Lip GY, Tse HF, Lane DA. Atrial Fibrillation. *Lancet*. 2012;379:648-661.
20. Fresco C, Proclemer A, on behalf of the PAFIT-2 Investigators. Management of recent onset atrial fibrillation. *Eur Heart J*. 1996;17(suppl C):C41-47.
21. Anderson JL, Gilbert EM, Alpert BL, et al. Flecainide Supraventricular Study Group. Prevention of symptomatic recurrences of paroxysmal atrial fibrillation in patients initially tolerating antiarrhythmic therapy. *Circulation*. 1989;80:1557-01570.
22. The Cardiac Arrhythmia Suppression Trial (CAST) Investigators. Preliminary report: effect of encainide and flecainide on mortality in a randomized trial of arrhythmia suppression after myocardial infarction. *N Engl J Med*. 1989;321:406-412.
23. Alboni P, Botto GL, Baldi N, et al. Outpatient treatment of recent-onset atrial fibrillation with the "pill-in-the-pocket" approach. *N Engl J Med*. 2004;351:2384-2391.
24. Hohnloser SH, Zabel M. Short and long term efficacy and safety of flecainide acetate for supraventricular arrhythmias. *Am J Cardiol*. 1992;70:3A-10A.
25. Leclercg JF, Chouty F, Denjoy I, et al. Flecainide in quinidine resistant atrial fibrillation. *Am J Cardiol*. 1992;70:62A-5A.
26. Antman EM, Beamer AD, Cautillon C, et al. Long term oral propafenone therapy for suppression of refractory symptomatic atrial fibrillation and atrial flutter. *J Am Coll Cardiol*. 1988;12:1005-1011.
27. Connolly SJ, Camm AJ, Halperin JL, et al; for the PALLAS Investigators. Dronedarone in highrisk permanent atrial fibrillation. *N Engl J Med*. 2011;365:2268-2276.
28. Vitolo E, Tronci M, Larovere MT, Rumolo R, Morabito A. Amiodarone versus quinidine in the prophylaxis of atrial fibrillation. *Acta Cardiol*. 1981;36:431-444.
29. Graboys TB, Podrid PJ, Lown B. Efficacy of amiodarone for refractory supraventricular tachyarrhythmias. *Am Heart J*. 1983;106:870-876.
30. Gosselink AM, Crijns HJ, Isabelle CVG, et al. Low dose amiodarone for maintenance of sinus rhythm after cardioversion of atrial fibrillation or atrial flutter. *JAMA*. 1992;267:3289-3293.
31. Acquati F, Forgione F, Caico S, et al. Prophylaxis of atrial fibrillation following electrical cardioversion. A prospective randomized study comparing low-dose and very low-dose amiodarone to propafenone: preliminary results (abstr). *J Am Coll Cardiol*. 1997;29:112A.

32. Gold RL, Haffajee CL, Charos G, et al. Amiodarone for refractory atrial fibrillation. *Am J Cardiol.* 1986;57:124-127.

33. Horowitz LN, Spielman SR, Greenspan AM, et al. Use of amiodarone in persistent and paroxysmal atrial fibrillation resistant to quinidine therapy. *J Am Coll Cardiol.* 1985;6:1402-1407.

34. Amiodarone Trials Meta-analysis Investigators. Effect of prophylactic amiodarone on mortality after acute myocardial infarction and in congestive heart failure: meta-analysis of individual data from 6500 patients in randomised trials. *Lancet.* 1997;350:1417–1424.

35. Lip GYH, Li-Saw-Hee FL. Paroxysmal atrial fibrillation. *Q J Med.* 2001;94:665–678.

36. Wann LS, Curtis AB, January CT, et al. 2011 ACCF/AHA/HRS focused update on the management of patients with atrial fibrillation (updating the 2006 guideline): a report of the American College of Cardiology Foundation/American Heart Association Task Force on Practice Guidelines. *Circulation.* 2011;123:104-123.

37. Umana E, Solares CA, Alpert MA. Tachycardia-induced cardiomyopathy. *Am J Med.* 2003;114:51-55.

38. Wann LS, Curtis AB, January CT, et al. 2011 ACCF/AHA/HRS focused update on the management of patients with atrial fibrillation (updating the 2006 guideline): a report of the American College of Cardiology Foundation/American Heart Association Task Force on Practice Guidelines. *Circulation.* 2011;123:104-123.

39. Royal College of Physicians of Edinburgh. Consensus Conference on Atrial Fibrillation: final consensus statement. *Proc R Coll Physicians Edin.* 1998;28:552-554.

40. Damiano RJ Jr, Gaynor SL, Bailey M, et al. The long-term outcome of patients with coronary disease and atrial fibrillation undergoing the Cox–Maze procedure. *J Thorac Cardiovasc Surg.* 2003;126:2016-2021.

41. Gillinov AM, McCarthy PM. Advances in the surgical treatment of atrial fibrillation. *Cardiol Clin.* 2004;22:147-157.

42. Stulak JM, Sundt TM IIIrd, Dearani JA, et al. Ten-year experience with the Cox–Maze procedure for atrial fibrillation: how do we define success? *Ann Thorac Surg.* 2007;83:1319-1324.

43. Stulak JM, Dearani JA, Sundt TM IIIrd, et al. Superiority of cut-and-sew technique for the Cox –Maze procedure: comparison with radiofrequency ablation. *J Thorac Cardiovasc Surg.* 2007;133:1022-1027.

44. Doty JR, Doty DB, Jones KW, et al. Comparison of standard Maze III and radiofrequency Maze operations for treatment of atrial fibrillation. *J Thorac Cardiovasc Surg.* 2007;133:1037-1044.

45. Gillinov AM. Advances in surgical treatment of atrial fibrillation. *Stroke.* 2007;38(part 2):618-623.

46. Natale A, Raviele A, Arentz T, et al. Venice Chart international consensus document on atrial fibrillation ablation. *J Cardiovasc Electrophysiol.* 2007;18:560-580.

47. Chen MS, Marrouche NF, Khaykin Y, et al. Pulmonary vein isolation for the treatment of atrial fibrillation in patients with impaired systolic function. *J Am Coll Cardiol.* 2004;43:1004-1009.

48. Wright M, Haïssaguerre M, Knecht S, et al. State of the art: catheter ablation of atrial fibrillation. *J Cardiovasc Electrophysiol.* 2008;19:583-592.

49. Hocini M, Sanders P, Jais P, et al. Techniques for curative treatment of atrial fibrillation. *J Cardiovasc Electrophysiol.* 2004;15:1467-1471.

50. Haissaguerre M, Sanders P, Hocini M, et al. Catheter ablation of long-lasting persistent atrial fibrillation: Critical structures for termination. *J Cardiovasc Electrophysiol.* 2005;16:1125-37.

51. Haissaguerre M, Hocini M, Sanders P, et al. Catheter ablation of long-lasting persistent atrial fibrillation: Clinical outcome and mechanisms of subsequent arrhythmias. *J Cardiovasc Electrophysiol.* 2005;16:1138-1147.

52. Cappato R, Calkins H, Chen SA, et al. Worldwide survey on the methods, efficacy, and safety of catheter ablation for human atrial fibrillation. *Circulation.* 2005;111:1100-1105.

53. Spragg DD, Dalal D, Cheema A, et al. Complications of catheter ablation for atrial fibrillation: incidence and predictors. *J Cardiovasc Electrophysiol*. 2008;19: 627-631.

Chapter 5

Anticoagulant treatment strategies for atrial fibrillation

A prothrombotic state is a characteristic of atrial fibrillation (AF), and the presence of AF is an independent risk factor for stroke and thromboembolism [1]. In accordance with the latest 2012 European Society of Cardiology (ESC) guidelines on AF, oral anticoagulation therapy should be considered in patients with AF who have one or more stroke risk factors [2]. The Congestive heart failure/left ventricular dysfunction, Hypertension, Age ≥75, Diabetes, Stroke (doubled) ($CHADS_2$) score is currently the most commonly used stroke risk stratification scheme and assigns points for heart failure, hypertension, age (≥75 years), diabetes, and history of stroke or transient ischemic attack (TIA) [2]. However, the ESC now recommend the Congestive heart failure/left ventricular dysfunction, Hypertension, Age ≥75 (doubled), Diabetes, Stroke (doubled) – Vascular disease, Age 65-74, and Sex category (female) (CHA_2DS_2-VASc) score, a modification of the $CHADS_2$, that also takes age (65–74 years), sex, and history of vascular disease (ie, previous myocardial infarction or peripheral arterial disease) into consideration to determine a patient's stroke risk [2,3]. Such a risk-scoring system identifies patients who are 'low-risk' (and thus will not benefit from anticoagulation therapy), and has been proven to be better than the $CHADS_2$ at identifying patients (both 'low risk' and 'high risk') who are likely to develop stroke and thromboembolism (Table 5.1) [4–6].

For patients with AF at risk of stroke (CHA_2DS_2-VASc ≥1), HAS-BLED (Hypertension, Abnormal renal/liver function, Stroke, Bleeding history or predisposition, Labile international normalized ratio, Elderly [>65 years], Drugs/alcohol concomitantly) score can help clinicians determine if use of anticoagulants outweighs the bleeding risk [2,7]. However, HAS-BLED scoring should not be used to exclude patients from receiving anticoagulants, but rather as a practical tool that can assist clinicians in making an informed treatment choice and highlighting possible correctible risk factors for bleeding (eg,

© Springer Healthcare 2014
Y.G. Yap and A.J. Camm, *Essentials of Atrial Fibrillation*,
DOI 10.1007/978-1-907673-98-6_5

Table 5.1 Assessment of stroke and bleeding risk			
CHA$_2$DS$_2$-VASc	Score	HAS-BLED	Score
Congestive heart failure /left ventricular dysfunction	1	Hypertension (SBP >160 mmHg)	1
Hypertension	1	Abnormal renal and liver function (1 point each)	1 or 2
Age ≥75 years	2	Stroke	1
Diabetes mellitus	1	Bleeding	1
Stroke/TIA/TE	2	Labile INRs	1
Vascular disease (prior MI, PAD or aortic plaque)	1	Elderly (e.g., age >65 years)	1
Age 65-74 years	1	Drugs or alcohol (1 point each)	1 or 2
Sex category (eg, female gender)	1		
Maximum score	9	Maximum score	9

CHA$_2$DS$_2$-VASc score of 0: recommend no antithrombotic therapy.
Score of 1: recommend antithrombotic therapy with oral anticoagulation or antiplatelet therapy (eg, when patients refuse oral anticoagulants), but preferably oral anticoagulation.
Score ≥2: recommend oral anticoagulation.
HAS-BLED score of ≥3 suggests increased bleeding risk and warrents some caution and/or regular review.

Table 5.1 Assessment of stroke and bleeding risk. CHA$_2$DS$_2$-VASc and HAS-BLED are two methods of assessing stroke and bleeding risk. CHA$_2$DS$_2$-VASc: Congestive heart failure/LV dysfunction, hypertension, aged ≥75 years (doubled), diabetes mellitus, prior stroke/TIA/ TE (doubled)-vascular disease, aged 65-74 years, sex category; HAS-BLED: Hypertension, abnormal renal/liver function, stroke, bleeding history or predisposition, labile INR, elderly (eg, >65 years of age), drugs/alcohol concomitantly; INR: International normalized ratio; MI: Myocardial infarction; PAD: Peripheral artery disease; SBP: Systolic blood pressure; TE: Thromboembolism; TIA: Transient ischemic attack.

controlling blood pressure, reducing use of non-steroidal anti-inflammatory drugs [2,7]. A proposed antithrombotic strategy for patients with AF is summarized in Figure 5.1 [2].

Generally, maximum protection against stroke in AF is achieved at an international normalized ratio (INR) range of 2.0–3.0, with a target of 2.5 being optimal for most patients with AF [8,9]. However, in patients with previous transient ischemic attack (TIA) or minor stroke, a higher range of 2.0–3.9 with a target of 3.0 may be used, although for those patients with higher risk of cerebral hemorrhage, a range of 1.6–2.5 with a target of 2.0 is sometimes recommended [9]. The INR should be determined at least weekly during initiation of treatment and monthly when stable [8].

In patients with AF and an acute stroke, cerebral imaging (CT or MRI) should be performed to exclude cerebral hemorrhage, and any uncontrolled

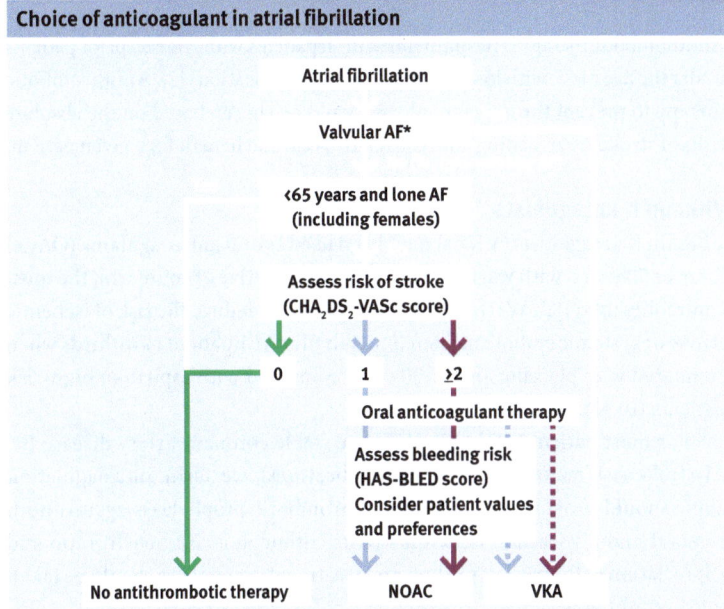

Figure 5.1 Choice of anticoagulant in atrial fibrillation. Antiplatelet therapy with aspirin plus clopidogrel, or – less effectively – aspirin only, should only be considered in patients who refuse OAC, or cannot tolerate OACs for reasons unrelated to bleeding. If there are contraindications to OAC or antiplatelet therapy, left atrial appendage occlusion, closure or excision may be considered. AF, atrial fibrillation; CHA$_2$DS$_2$-VASc, Congestive heart failure/left ventricular dysfunction, Hypertension, Age ≥75 (doubled), Diabetes, Stroke (doubled) – Vascular disease, Age 65-74, and Sex category (female); HAS-BLED, Hypertension, Abnormal renal/liver function, Stroke, Bleeding history or predisposition, Labile international normalized ratio, Elderly (>65 years), Drugs/alcohol concomitantly; NOAC, novel oral anticoagulant; OAC, oral anticoagulant; VKA, vitamin K agonist. *Includes rheumatic valvular disease and mechanical prosthetic valves. Reproduced with permission from Camm et al [2].

hypertension should be appropriately treated. In the absence of hemorrhage, anticoagulation therapy should begin only after 2 weeks, but if hemorrhage is present, anticoagulation therapy should not be given [10]. If the patient has had a large cerebral infarction, the initiation of anticoagulation therapy should be delayed. Similarly, in patients with AF and an acute TIA, imaging (CT or MRI) should be performed to exclude recent cerebral infarction or hemorrhage and, if so, anticoagulation therapy should begin as soon as possible [8].

Antithrombotic therapy in atrial fibrillation

Antithombotic therapy is recommended in all patients with AF, except for patients under the age of 65, with lone AF, or with contraindications [2]. Antithrombotic therapy to prevent thromboembolism should be chosen based on the absolute risks of stroke and bleeding, and the relative risk and benefit for a given patient.

Vitamin K antagonists

Vitamin K antagonists (VKAs) have been used as oral anticoagulants (OACs) for over 50 years, with warfarin, a synthetic derivative of coumarin, the most commonly used [11]. Warfarin has been proven to reduce the risk of ischemic stroke or systemic embolism from non-valvular AF by about two-thirds when compared with placebo, and by 30–40% compared with aspirin in high-risk patients [10,12].

For most patients with AF who have stable coronary artery disease (ie, ≥1 stroke risk factor with no contraindications), warfarin anticoagulation alone should provide satisfactory antithrombotic prophylaxis against both cerebral and myocardial ischemic events, although a risk-benefit ratio and appreciation of the patient's values and treatment preferences should be taken into account [8,9].

Antiplatelet therapy

In the past, antiplatelet therapy with aspirin (75–325 mg/daily) alone has been used in patients who are at low risk of embolic stroke, such as young patients (aged <65 years) who have no history of hypertension, cerebral vascular disease, congestive heart failure, or diabetes [9]. However, now aspirin alone, or in combination with clopidogrel is now recommended in patients for whom VKAs are contraindicated, in patients who refuse OACs, or in those that cannot tolerate OACs due to contraindications unrelated to bleeding [2].

Several studies have explored the prophylactic effects of antiplatelet therapy, most commonly aspirin compared with placebo, on the risk of thromboembolism in patients with AF. In a meta-analysis by Hart and colleagues, treatment with aspirin was associated with a nonsignificant 19% (95% CI –1% to –35%) reduction in the incidence of stroke [11]. The beneficial effect of aspirin monotherapy was driven by the results of one positive study, SPAF-I, which showed a 42% stroke risk reduction with aspirin versus placebo [13]. However, aspirin was ineffective in patients older than 75 years and did not prevent severe or recurrent strokes. The SPAF-I trial was also stopped early and its result may be exaggerated.

Oral anticoagulants were superior to the combination of aspirin plus clopidogrel in the preventing of vascular events in a large trial (6706 patients; relative risk [RR] reduction 40%; 95% CI, 18–56%) [14]. Similarly, there was no advantage in all-cause mortality or in the composite of stroke (ischemic and hemorrhagic), myocardial infarction, or vascular death, with the combination of aspirin and clopidogrel compared with aspirin alone in patients with a history of AF and stable cardiovascular disease or multiple cardiovascular risk factors [15]. Recent evidence has demonstrated that the combination of clopidogrel and aspirin substantially reduces the ischemic stroke rate compared with aspirin treatment alone in patients with AF who are resistant to or intolerant of VKAs [16]. However, antiplatelet therapy has not been proven to be safer when compared to warfarin (especially in the elderly), and is now generally considered an inferior strategy for stroke prevention in AF [17].

Novel oral anticoagulants

Novel oral anticoagulant drugs (NOACs) are poised to replace warfarin as effective anticoagulants for the prevention of strokes in patients with AF. In contrast to VKAs, which inhibit the formation of multiple active vitamin K-dependent coagulation factors, these drugs block the activity of a single step in the coagulation cascade and have no requirement for coagulation monitoring. Two categories of oral anticoagulants, oral factor Xa inhibitors (eg, rivaroxaban, apixaban, and edoxaban) and direct thrombin inhibitors (dabigatran), have recently been approved or are in clinical development. All of these agents appear to be effective [18]. NOACs are considered broadly preferable to VKA in the majority of patients with non-valvular AF, with strict adherence to approved indications [2].

Direct factor Xa inhibitors

Several new factor Xa inhibitors are in development or have recently been approved for thromboprophylaxis in AF, including apixaban, rivaroxaban and edoxaban.

Apixaban

During the AVERROES trial, apixaban was found to be an efficacious treatment for patients at high risk of stroke who were unsuitable for (or unwilling to take) vitamin K antagonist therapy (eg, warfarin) [19]. The primary outcome of this double-blind, Phase III, randomized study was the occurrence of stroke or systemic embolism; of the 5599 randomly assigned patients with AF, there were 51 primary outcome events (1.6% per year) among patients assigned to apixaban 5 mg twice daily and 113 (3.7% per year) among those assigned to 81–324 mg of aspirin per day (HR=0.45; 95% CI, 0.32–0.62; $P<0.001$). Furthermore, aspirin was significantly less well tolerated than apixaban, as indicated by the rate of permanent discontinuations ($P=0.03$) [19].

Additionally, the ARISTOTLE trial demonstrated that apixaban (5 mg twice daily) was superior to warfarin in preventing stroke and systemic embolism [20]. The randomized, double-blind study involved 18,201 patients with atrial fibrillation and at least one additional risk factor for stroke. There was a significant reduction in the primary efficacy outcome (rate of stroke or systemic embolism) with apixaban: 1.27% per year compared with 1.60% per year in the warfarin group (HR=0.79; 95% CI, 0.66–0.95; $P<0.001$ for noninferiority and $P=0.01$ for superiority [a secondary efficacy analysis]). Reductions in major bleeding (31%) and all-cause mortality (but not cardiovascular mortality; 11%) were also observed with apixaban compared with warfarin [20].

In November 2012, the European Medicines Agency approved apixaban for the prevention of stroke and thromboembolism in adults with non-valvular AF and one or more risk factors, followed shortly afterwards by FDA approval in December 2012.

Rivaroxaban

The landmark ROCKET-AF trial, a prospective, randomized, double-blind, double-dummy parallel group outcomes study, compared once-daily rivaroxaban (20 mg, or 15 mg for patients with moderate renal impairment) with dose-adjusted warfarin in 14,264 patients with non-valvular AF who were at moderate-to-high risk for stroke or non-CNS systemic embolism for whom the major guidelines recommend anticoagulation [21]. In ROCKET-AF, treatment with once-daily rivaroxaban demonstrated noninferiority in preventing stroke and systemic embolism versus warfarin (HR=0.79; 95% CI, 0.66 to 0.96; $P<0.001$ for noninferiority) [21]. The principal safety outcome – the composite of major and non-major clinically relevant bleeding events – was similar in both the rivaroxaban and warfarin groups (14.9%/year and 14.5%/year, respectively; HR=1.03; 95% CI, 0.96 to 1.11; $P=0.44$). Rates of major bleeding were also similar between the groups [21]. Importantly, patients on rivaroxaban suffered significantly less bleeding into a critical organ (rivaroxban [0.8%/ year] versus warfarin [1.2%/year]; $P=0.007$) or fatal bleeding (0.2%/year versus 0.5%/year; $P=0.003$), and significantly fewer intracranial hemorrhages (0.5%/ year versus 0.7%/year; $P=0.02$), while decreases in hemoglobin levels of ≥2 g/dL (2.8%/year vs 2.3%/year; P=0.02) and transfusions (1.6%/year vs. 1.3%/ year; P=0.04) were more common with rivaroxaban when compared with warfarin [21]. In the Japanese ROCKET-AF (J-ROCKET AF) trial of 1280 patients with non-valvular AF at a high risk for stroke, rivaroxaban was non-inferior to warfarin with respect to the primary safety outcome (a composite of major and nonmajor clinically relevant bleeding events). The rate of the primary safety outcome was 18.0%/year in rivaroxaban-treated patients and 16.4%/year in warfarin-treated patients (HR=1.11; 95% CI, 0.87–1.42; $P<0.001$ for non-inferiority) [22].

Rivaroxaban has been shown to have a reassuring cardiovascular profile with no increase in myocardial infarctions or dyspepsia [23]. Also, the efficacy of rivaroxaban when compared with warfarin was consistent among patients with previous stroke or TIA (HR=0.94, 95% CI, 0.77–1.16), as well as in those without a history of stroke or TIA (HR=0.77, 95% CI, 0.58–1.01; $P=0.23$ for the interaction of treatment) [23].

Special consideration should be taken with patients with renal dysfunction, as they are at higher risk of stroke, systemic embolism, and bleeding, regardless of treatment [24]. In ROCKET-AF, patients with moderate renal dysfunction (creatinine clearance 30-49 mL/min) received 15 mg rivaroxaban once daily instead of 20 mg rivaroxaban or dose-adjusted warfarin [21]. Among those with moderate renal dysfunction, stroke or systemic embolism (the primary endpoint) occurred in 2.32%/year with rivaroxaban 15 mg/day, compared to 2.77 with warfarin [HR=0.84; 95% CI, 0.57–1.23]. Additionally, rates of major and clinically relevant non-major bleeding and intracranial bleeding were similar with rivaroxaban or warfarin [21].

At the end of 2011, rivaroxaban received marketing approval in the US and the EU for use in prevention of stroke and systemic embolism in patients with nonvalvular AF with one or more risk factors.

Edoxaban

Edoxaban is currently in development for the reduction of risk in stroke or systemic embolic events in patients with AF. A dose-ranging, parallel-group, multicenter, multinational, Phase II trial randomized 1146 patients with AF to receive once- or twice-daily edoxaban (30 mg or 60 mg) or warfarin [25]. Once-daily treatment with edoxaban caused less bleeding than treatment with warfarin; however, twice-daily dosing caused more bleeding. All treatment groups had similar bilirubin values and hepatic enzyme levels [25].

Another Phase II study was conducted in 536 Japanese patients with non-valvular AF. Patients were randomized to receive warfarin, adjusted to a target prothrombin time, or edoxaban 30, 45, or 60 mg once daily [26]. The number of bleeding events was higher in those taking edoxaban 60 mg than in those taking warfarin, but lower in those taking edoxaban 30 mg. However, there were no significant differences in bleeding between the edoxaban groups or between any edoxaban group and the warfarin group. Only one thromboembolic event was noted, in a patient taking edoxaban 45 mg [26].

The ongoing Phase III ENGAGE-AF trial is comparing the efficacy and safety of edoxaban (30 mg or 60 mg once daily) with warfarin in patients with a documented history of AF during the past year and a moderate-to-high stroke risk (CHADS$_2$ score ≥2)[27]. Patients will be followed for a minimum of 24 months; the primary efficacy endpoint is the composite of stroke and systemic embolic events. The safety endpoint is major bleeding events. An estimated 21,105 patients have been enrolled in this study [27].

Direct thrombin inhibitors
Dabigitran etexilate
Dabigatran etexilate is an oral prodrug that is rapidly converted by a serum esterase to dabigatran, a potent, direct, competitive inhibitor of thrombin. The RE-LY trial evaluated the effect of dabigatran compared with warfarin in 18,113 patients with AF [28]. This was a randomized, open-label, Phase III trial, comparing two blinded doses of dabigatran (110 mg or 150 mg twice daily) with open-label adjusted-dose warfarin. Dabigatran 110 mg twice daily was associated with rates of stroke and systemic embolism that were similar to those associated with warfarin (relative risk [RR] with dabigatran, 0.91; 95% CI, 0.74–1.11; $P<0.001$ for non-inferiority), as well as lower rates of major hemorrhage (2.71%/year vs 3.36%/year; $P=0.003$) [28]. Lower rates of stroke and systemic embolism were seen with dabigatran 150 mg compared with warfarin (RR with dabigatran, 0.66; 95% CI, 0.53–0.82; $P<0.001$ for superiority) but the rates of major hemorrhage were similar (3.11%/year vs 3.36%/year; $P=0.31$). While rates of hemorrhagic stroke and intracranial bleeding were significantly lower with both doses of dabigatran, a significantly higher rate of major gastrointestinal bleeding was observed with dabigatran 150 mg when compared with warfarin [28].

The mortality rate in RE-LY was 4.13%/year in the warfarin group, 3.75%/year in the dabigatran 110 mg group ($P=0.13$), and 3.64%/year in the dabigatran 150 mg group ($P=0.051$) [28]. Based on the results of RE-LY, dabigatran was approved for prevention of stroke and systemic embolism in the US (150 mg twice daily; 75 mg twice daily in those with severe renal impairment) and EU (for patients with non-valvular AF with at least one risk factor; both 110 mg and 150 mg twice daily doses approved), as well as in many countries worldwide.

Clinical application

The NOACs (apixaban, rivaroxaban, and dabigatran) have been shown to be non-inferior to VKAs for a majority of patients with non-valvular AF [2]. However, it is crucial that when treating patients with NOACs, adherence to approved indications must be enforced, as evidence and experience in their use remains limited. According to a recent meta-analyses, no major differences in safety and efficacy between NOACs have been found [29].

Special considerations

Careful consideration in the prevention of thrombotic or thromboembolic events must be taken in patients that have undergone a recent percutaneous coronary intervention (PCI) with stent placement, particularly with a drug-eluting stent [30]. It is known that the concomitant use of antiplatelet therapy with OACs significantly increases the risk of bleeding and has been associated with major bleeding rates as high as 7% [31]. Patients with AF who have more than one moderate risk factor for thromboembolism (clinical heart failure or impaired left ventricular systolic function [ejection fraction $\leq$ 35%], history of hypertension, age >75 years, diabetes mellitus, prior stroke, or TIA score $\geq$ 2) should resume anticoagulation as soon as feasible after PCI [30]. For those at low risk of serious bleeding, treatment with triple therapy may be the best option [30].

In patients with AF who have risk factors for thromboembolism requiring chronic anticoagulation, a bare-metal stent may be preferable to drug-eluting stents in order to reduce the need for prolonged combination therapy [31–33]. Large, randomized, prospective studies are required to assess the bleeding and thrombotic risk with various post-PCI strategies in order to facilitate the development of guidelines.

Left atrial appendage occlusion devices that prevent thromboembolism from the left atrial appendage are under development.

References

1. Watson T, Shantsila E, Lip GY. Mechanisms of thrombogenesis in atrial fibrillation: Virchow's triad revisited.. *Lancet.* 2009;373:155-66.
2. Camm AJ, Lip GYH, De Caterina R, et al. 2012 focused update of the ESC Guidelines for the management of atrial fibrillation. An update of the 2010 ESC Guidelines for the management of atrial fibrillation. *Eur Heart J.* 2012;33:2719-2747.
3. Coppens M, Eikelboom JW, Hart RG, et al. The CHA_2DS_2-VASc score identifies those patients with atrial fibrillation and a CHADS2 score of 1 who are unlikely to benefit from oral anticoagulant therapy. *Eur Heart J.* 2013;34:170-176.

4. Friberg L, Rosenqvist M, Lip GY. Evaluation of risk stratification schemes for ischaemic stroke and bleeding in 182 678 patients with atrial fibrillation: the Swedish Atrial Fibrillation cohort study. *Eur Heart J*. 2012;33:1500-1510.
5. Olesen JB, Lip GY, Hansen ML, et al. Validation of risk stratification schemes for predicting stroke and thromboembolism in patients with atrial fibrillation: nationwide cohort study. *Br Med J*. 2011;3:42.
6. Boriani G, Botto GL, Padeletti L, et al; Italian AT-500 Registry Investigators. Improving stroke risk stratification using the CHADS$_2$ and CHA$_2$DS$_2$-VASc risk scores in patients with paroxysmal atrial fibrillation by continuous arrhythmia burden monitoring. *Stroke*. 2011;42:1768-1770.
7. Pisters R, Lane DA, Nieuwlaat R, de Vos CB, Crijns HJ, Lip GY. A novel user-friendly score (HAS-BLED) to assess 1-year risk of major bleeding in patients with atrial fibrillation: the Euro Heart Survey. *Chest*. 2010;138:1093-1100.
8. Fuster V, Rydén LE, Cannom DS, et al. 2011 ACCF/AHA/HRS focused updates incorporated into the ACC/AHA/ESC 2006 guidelines for the management of patients with atrial fibrillation: a report of the American College of Cardiology Foundation/American Heart Association Task Force on practice guidelines. Circulation. 2011;123:e269-e367.
9. Cairns JA. Atrial fibrillation: antithrombotic therapy. In,Yusuf S, Cairns JA, Camm AJ, Fallen EL, Gersh BJ, eds. *Evidence Based Cardiology*. London: BMJ Books, 1998:544-552.
10. Aguilar MI, Hart R, Pearce LA. Oral anticoagulants versus antiplatelet therapy for preventing stroke in patients with non-valvular atrial fibrillation and no history of stroke or transient ischemic attacks. *Cochrane Database Syst Rev*. 2007;3:CD006186.
11. Hart RG, Pearce LA, Aguilar MI. Meta-analysis: antithrombotic therapy to prevent stroke in patients who have nonvalvular atrial fibrillation. *Ann Intern Med*. 2007;146:857-867.
12. Lip GY, Edwards SJ. Stroke prevention with aspirin, warfarin and ximelagatran in patients with non-valvular atrial fibrillation: a systemic review and meta-analysis. *Thromb Res*. 2006;118:321-333.
13. Stroke prevention in Atrial Fibrillation (SPAF) Investigators. A differential effect of aspirin in prevention of stroke on atrial fibrillation. *J Stroke Cerebrovasc Dis*. 1993;3:181-188.
14. Connolly S, Pogue J, Hart R, et al. Clopidogrel plus aspirin versus oral anticoagulation for atrial fibrillation in the Atrial fibrillation Clopidogrel Trial with Irbesartan for prevention of Vascular Events (ACTIVE W): a randomised controlled trial. *Lancet*. 2006;367:1903-1912.
15. Hart RG, Bhatt DL, Hacke W, et al CHARISMA Investigators. Clopidogrel and aspirin versus aspirin alone for the prevention of stroke in patients with a history of atrial fibrillation: subgroup analysis of the CHARISMA randomized trial. *Cerebrovasc Dis*. 2008;25:344-347.
16. The ACTIVE Investigators. Effect of clopidogrel added to aspirin in patients with atrial fibrillation. N Engl J Med. 2009;360:2066-2078.
17. Lip GY. The role of aspirin for stroke prevention in atrial fibrillation. *Nat Rev Cardiol*. 2011;8:602-606.
18. Contractor T, Levin V, Martinez MW, Marchlinski FE. Novel oral anticoagulants for stroke prevention in patients with atrial fibrillation: dawn of a new era. *Postgrad Med*. 2013;125:34-44.
19. Connolly SJ, Eikelboom J, Joyner C, et al; for the AVERROES Steering Committee and Investigators. Apixaban in patients with atrial fibrillation. *N Engl J Med*. 2011;364:806-817.
20. Granger CB, Alexander JH, McMurray JJV, et al; for the ARISTOTLE Committees and Investigators. Apixaban versus warfarin in patients with atrial fibrillation. *N Engl J Med* 2011;365:981-992.
21. Patel MR, Mahaffey KW, Garg J, et al; for the ROCKET AF Investigators. Rivaroxaban versus warfarin in nonvalvular atrial fibrillation. *N Engl J Med*. 2011;365:883-891.

22. Hori M, Matsumoto M, Tanahashi N, et al; on behalf of J-ROCKET AF study investigators. Rivaroxaban vs. warfarin in Japanese patients with atrial fibrillation – the J-ROCKET AF study. *Circ J*. 2012;76:2104-2111.
23. Hankey GJ, Patel MR, Stevens SR, et al. Rivaroxaban compared with warfarin in patients with atrial fibrillation and previous stroke or transient ischaemic attack: a subgroup analysis of ROCKET AF. *Lancet Neurol*. 2012;11:315-322.
24. Fox KAA, Piccini JP, Wojdyla D, et al. Prevention of stroke and systemic embolism with rivaroxaban compared with warfarin in patients with non-valvular atrial fibrillation and moderate renal impairment. *Eur Heart J*. 2011;32:2387-2394.
25. Weitz JI, Connolly SJ, Patel I, et al. Randomised, parallel-group, multicentre, multinational phase 2 study comparing edoxaban, an oral factor Xa inhibitor, with warfarin for stroke prevention in patients with atrial fibrillation. *Thromb Haemost*. 2010;104:633-641.
26. Yamashita T, Koretsune Y, Yasaka M, et al. Randomized, multicenter, warfarin-controlled Phase II study of edoxaban in Japanese patients with non-valvular atrial fibrillation. *Circ J*. 2012;76:1840-1847.
27. ClinicalTrials.gov Website. A phase 3, randomized, double-blind, double-dummy, parallel group, multi-center, multi-national study for evaluation of efficacy and safety of edoxaban (DU-176b) versus warfarin in subjects with atrial fibrillation - Effective Anticoagulation With Factor Xa Next Generation in Atrial Fibrillation (ENGAGE-AF TIMI-48). http://clinicaltrials.gov/ct/show/NCT00781391. Accessed September 12, 2013.
28. Connolly SJ, Ezekowitz MD, Yusuf S, et al; for the RE-LY Steering Committee and Investigators. Dabigatran versus warfarin in patients with atrial fibrillation. *N Engl J Med*. 2009;361:1139-1151.
29. Lip GY, Larsen TB, Skjøth F, Rasmussen LH. Indirect comparisons of new oral anticoagulant drugs for efficacy and safety when used for stroke prevention in atrial fibrillation. *J Am Coll Cardiol*. 2012;60:738-746.
30. Camm AJ, Kirchhof P, Lip GYH, et al. Guidelines for the management of atrial fibrillationThe Task Force for the Management of Atrial Fibrillation of the European Society of Cardiology (ESC). *Europace*. 2010;12:1360-1420.
31. Pengo V, Legnani C, Noventa F, Palareti G; for the ISCOAT Study Group. Italian Study on Complications of Oral Anticoagulant Therapy. Oral anticoagulant therapy in patients with nonrheumatic atrial fibrillation and risk of bleed. A multicenter inception cohort study. *Thromb Haemost*. 2001;85:418-22.
32. Lip GY, Karpha M. Anticoagulant and antiplatelet therapy use in patients with atrial fibrillation undergoing percutaneous coronary intervention: the need for consensus and a management guideline. *Chest*. 2006;130:1823-1827.
33. Nguyen MC, Murphy SA, Mega JL, et al. Triple therapy (TTx): ASA, thienopyridine and oral anticoagulation (OA) therapy following ST elevation myocardial infarction (STEMI): is it safe? (abstract 2221). *Circulation*. 2007;116(suppl II):II-483.